Fluids and Electrolytes

*A fast and easy way to understand
acid-base balance without memorization*

Dr. Gabriel J. Connor

Table of Contents

Introduction

Sodium, potassium, and their related anions are essential elements of all body fluids. Sodium is the main cation of intracellular fluid and potassium. Complex pathways control the amounts of electrolytes in body fluids and the volume of both the extracellular and intracellular fluid compartments. Processes that sustain gradient concentrations of these cations through cell membranes require energy; at least three transport mechanisms tend to be involved. Regulation of fluid volumes and concentrations affects the cardiovascular and endocrine systems, the central nervous system, and the autonomic nervous system; they all function mainly by controlling the rate at which water and electrolytes are excreted by the kidneys.

Archaeological and anthropological findings indicate that hunter-gatherers' diets during the Paleolithic period and the diet of today's traditional cultures outside the mainstream community have, with few exceptions, high potassium levels, and very low sodium levels. Salt has traditionally been rare in most regions, and has been highly regarded by early humans and many ancient civilizations in Asia, Africa, and Europe. It has been used in ceremonies and for the storage of food in many primitive cultures. A mechanism for maintaining extracellular fluid volume in the face of dehydration, trauma, hemorrhage, breastfeeding, and lactation may be biologically beneficial in areas of lack of salt. The physiology of mammals has thus developed to facilitate salt storage in the kidneys, gastrointestinal tract, and sweat glands, and establish a taste for sodium chloride in the brain's tongue-and-salt appetite.

There is evidence of salt-appetite centers in the central nervous system in some animals, and there is a reason for the taste of salt in humans and many mammals. Salt-appetite occurs during acute salt deficiency and hypovolemia. The latest research indicates that there are two levels of salt-appetite: the physiological level of salt consumption required to sustain body fluid volume and to maintain adequate arterial pressure on the blood-vessel tissues; and the higher range of salt-appetite, which is dictated by a learned urge to eat salt above physiological requirements. Deprivation of these higher salt levels has resulted in a preference for less salt for many months.

Neolithic farming communities also evolved numerous methods of food processing and storage. Salt is typically used for meat and dairy products. Most modem processing processes, including grain processing and processed flours, increase sodium content and decrease potassium, whether or not required for preservation. During meal processing, more salt is applied to the menu, and salt is available on the table itself.

The following book is a humble effort to explain these important components of our life. There is detail about normal mechanisms to regulate fluid and electrolytes in the body, how different diseases cause their imbalance, brief details about how to manage them clinically, and most importantly, how to memorize important aspects. In the end, there are a few practice questions as well to test your understanding of the concepts.

Chapter 1
Basic Concepts

Solute and Solvent
These are the components of a solution: The dissolving substance is called a solvent, while the dissolved substance is called a solute or a substance (usually in a lesser amount) dissolved in a new substance. A classic example of a solution is sugar dissolved in water: sugar is the solute, and water is the solvent.

Osmolarity
By definition, osmolarity is the measure of solute concentration per unit VOLUME of solvent. Osmolarity considers ALL of the solute concentrations, not just those that cannot cross the semipermeable membrane.

Osmolality
Osmolality is defined as the measure of solute concentration per unit MASS of solvent. We never measure osmolarity in practice because water changes its volume according to temperature (but the mass remains the same) Osmolality is the same in both the ICF and the ECF. Equally inside and outside of the cell, the osmolality is 285-290 mOsm/Kg.

Tonicity
Tonicity is the assessment of the osmotic pressure gradient between the two solutions. Unlike osmolarity, tonicity is only affected by solutes that cannot cross this semipermeable membrane, and they are the only solutes that affect the osmotic pressure gradient. So, you can have iso-osmolar solutions that are not isotonic. The major "effective" osmole is SODIUM. Sodium and its associated anions contribute to 86% of the osmolality and 92% of the tonicity.

Isotonic

Iso: Same/Equal Tonic: concentration of a solution. The cell has almost the same concentration inside and outside that under normal conditions, and the intracellular and extracellular cells are both isotonic. Examples of Isotonic fluids are:
- 0.9% Saline
- 5% Dextrose in saline of 0.225% (D5W1/4NS)
- 5% Dextrose in water (D5W).

Isotonic fluids are used to raise EXTRACELLULAR fluid's quantity due to blood loss, surgery, vomiting, or dehydration leading to extracellular loss of fluid.

Hypotonic

Hypo: under/beneath. Tonic: concentration of a solution. The cell has a low quantity of extracellular solute and it needs to be moved into the cell to bring it back to normal through osmosis. This would otherwise cause CELL SWELLING, which can cause the cell to burst or lyse.
Examples of Hypotonic solutions

- 0.45% Saline (1/2 NS)
- 0.225% Saline (1/4 NS)
- 0.33% saline (1/3 NS)

Hypotonic solutions are used where the cell is dehydrated, and fluids need to be returned intracellularly. This develops as patients experience diabetic ketoacidosis (DKA) or hyperosmolar hyperglycemia. Important: Look out for the loss of the fluid from the circulatory system when you attempt to rehydrate extracellular fluid in a patient. Never offer hypotonic solutions to patients at risk of elevated cranial pressure (may allow fluid to transfer to brain tissue), extreme burns, trauma (already hypovolemic), etc., so the fluid volume may be reduced.

Hypertonic

Hyper: excessive. Tonic: concentration of a solution. The cell has an excessive volume of solute extracellularly, and the osmosis allows water to flow out of the cell from intracellular space to the extracellular space, which causes CELL TO SHRINK.

Examples of Hypertonic solutions
- 3% Saline
- 5% Saline
- 5% Dextrose in 0.9% Saline
- 5% Dextrose in 0.45% saline
- 5% Dextrose in Lactated Ringer's
- 10% Dextrose in Water (D10W)

Hypertonic solutions are used very carefully. They are more likely to be provided in the ICU due to the sudden side effects of pulmonary edema/fluid overload). Hypertonic solutions are often given through the central venous line.

Types of Solutions

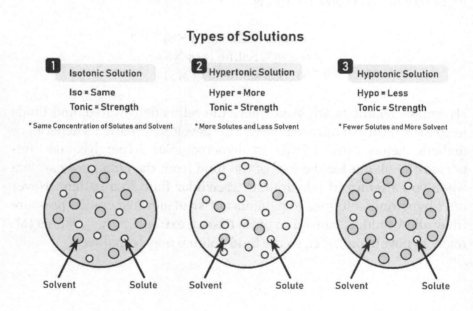

1 Isotonic Solution
Iso = Same
Tonic = Strength
*Same Concentration of Solutes and Solvent
Solvent   Solute

2 Hypertonic Solution
Hyper = More
Tonic = Strength
*More Solutes and Less Solvent
Solvent   Solute

3 Hypotonic Solution
Hypo = Less
Tonic = Strength
*Fewer Solutes and More Solvent
Solvent   Solute

Chapter 2
Body Fluids

As stated, the major body fluid is water. In a lean individual, it comprises about 60% of the total body weight. Fat contains a reduced amount of water. Therefore, in obese individuals, the water content is about 55% of the total body weight. For example, a 70 kg lean person contains 42 L of water (70 × 0.6 = 42 L).

Body Fluid Compartments
The total body water is distributed between two major compartments: the *extracellular fluid* (ECF) and *intracellular fluid* (ICF) compartments. About one-third of the total amount of water (20% of body weight) is confined to the ECF and two-thirds of the water (40% of body weight) to the ICF compartment. The ECF compartment, in turn, is divided into the following subdivisions:
- Plasma
- Interstitial fluid and lymph
- Bone and dense connective tissue water
- Transcellular (cerebrospinal, pleural, peritoneal, synovial, and digestive secretions).
In this subdivision, the plasma and interstitial fluids are the two most important because of the constant fluid and electrolyte exchange. The capillary endothelium separates plasma and interstitial fluid. Plasma circulates in the blood vessels, whereas the interstitial fluid bathes all tissue cells except for the formed blood elements.
Intracellular Fluid
The intracellular fluid (or cytoplasm) is the fluid that is found within the cells. It is divided into compartments by membranes that encircle the various organelles of the cell. For instance, the mitochondrial matrix divides the mitochondria into compartments.
The eukaryotic cell contents inside the cell membrane, except the cell nucleus and other membrane-bound organelles (e.g. mitochondria, endoplasmic reticulum lumen, etc.), are referred to as cytoplasm.

Extracellular Fluid

Extracellular fluid (ECF), also known as extracellular fluid volume (ECFV), typically signifies all body fluids outside the cells. Extracellular fluid can be classified into two main subdivisions: interstitial fluid and blood plasma. The extracellular fluid also contains the transcellular fluid, which makes up just about 2.5 percent of the ECF. The standard glucose concentration in extracellular fluid controlled by homeostasis in humans is approximately 5 mM per L. The pH of the extracellular fluid is closely regulated by the buffers and is retained at about 7.4. The ECF volume is normally 15L (12L of interstitial fluid and 3L of plasma). The ECF includes extracellular matrices (ECMs) that serve as suspension fluids for cells and molecules inside the ECF.

Blood Plasma

Blood plasma is a straw-colored/pale-yellow liquid portion of blood that usually keeps blood cells in suspension, rendering it a form of ECM for blood cells and a diverse group of molecules. It is around 55% of the overall blood volume. It is the intravascular fluid portion of the extracellular fluid. It is mainly water (93% by volume) and includes dissolved proteins (the primary proteins are fibrinogens, globulins, and albumins), clotting factors, glucose, mineral ions ($Na+$, $Ca++$, $Mg++$, $HCO3-Cl-$, etc.), hormones, and carbon dioxide (plasma is the key medium for excretory substance transport). It plays a crucial role in intravascular osmotic effects that keep electrolyte levels regulated and protect the body from infection and other blood conditions.

Interstitial Fluid

Interstitial fluid (or tissue fluid) is a liquid that bathes and covers the cells in multicellular organisms. Interstitial fluid is present in interstitial areas, also known as tissue spaces. On average, a human has about 11 liters (2.4 imperial gallons or about 2.9 US gal.) of interstitial fluid that provides the body with nutrients and waste disposal. The bulk of the interstitial space behaves as an ECM, and the fluid space consists of cell-excreted molecules that lie between the basement membranes of the interstitial spaces. Interstitial ECM includes several connective tissues and proteins (such as collagen) implicated in blood clotting and wound recovery.

Transcellular Fluid

The transcellular fluid is the fraction of total body water in epithelial-lined spaces. It is the smallest portion of extracellular fluid, compared to the interstitial fluid and plasma. It is also not measured as a percentage of the extracellular fluid, as much as 2.5 percent of the total body water. Examples of this fluid include the cerebrospinal fluid, the ocular fluid, the joint fluid, and the pleural cavity containing fluid in their respective epithelial-lined spaces. The transcellular fluid function is mainly the lubrication of these cavities and often the transport of electrolytes.

Body Fluid Composition

The tissue fluid-structure depends on the interaction between the cells in the biological tissue and the blood. This means that the distribution of fluids differs between the body compartments.

Intracellular Fluid Composition

Cytosol or intracellular fluid consists primarily of water, dissolved ions, small molecules, and large, water-soluble molecules (such as proteins). This combination of small molecules is highly complex since the number of enzymes involved in cell metabolism is enormous. These enzymes are active in biochemical pathways that help cells and activate or deactivate toxins. The bulk of cytosols is water, which makes up around 70% of the total volume of a normal cell. The pH of the intracellular fluid should be 7.4. The cell membrane divides the cytosol from the extracellular fluid but can there can be movement across the membrane through specialized channels and pumps during passive and active transport. The other ions in the intracellular fluid are somewhat different from those in the extracellular fluid. Cytosol also contains significantly larger concentrations of charged macromolecules such as proteins and nucleic acids than outside the cell. Compared to extracellular fluid, cytosol has a high concentration of potassium ions and a low sodium ion concentration. These sodium and potassium ion concentrations are responsible for the $Na+/K$ ATPase pumps that promote these ions' active transport. These pumps transport ions toward their concentration gradients to preserve the cytosol fluid structure of the ions.

Extracellular Fluid Composition

Extracellular fluid is predominantly in the form of cations and anions. Cations consist of sodium (Na+ = 136–145 mEq/L), potassium (K+ = 3.5–5.5 mEq/L) and calcium (Ca2+ = 8.4–10.5 mEq/L). Anions include chloride (mEq/L) and carbonate hydrogen (HCO3- 22-26 mM). These ions are essential for the transport of water in the body. Plasma is mainly water (93 percent by volume) and includes dissolved proteins (the largest proteins being fibrinogens, globulins, and albumins), glucose, clotting agents, mineral ions (Na+, Ca++, Mg++, HCO3-, Cl-, etc.), hormones, and carbon dioxide (plasma is the primary source for excretory substance transport). These dissolved compounds are involved in several biochemical processes, such as gas exchange, immune system activity, and drug delivery within the body.

Transcellular Fluid Composition

Owing to the various situations, the composition of transcellular fluid varies significantly. Four of the electrolytes in the transcellular fluid are sodium ions, chloride ions, and bicarbonate ions. Cerebrospinal fluid is similar to blood plasma, although it lacks most proteins, such as albumin since it is too large to get across the blood-brain barrier. Ocular fluid in the eyes compares with cerebrospinal fluid by having high protein quantities, including antibodies.

Fluid Movement

Membranes segregate the extracellular fluid from the main compartments of the body. These membranes are hydrophobic and restrain water; however, there are a few ways fluids can travel between body compartments. There are small openings in membranes, such as close junctions, which cause fluids and some of their contents to move through membranes through pressure gradients.

Formation of Interstitial Fluid

The pumping of the heart gives rise to hydrostatic pressure during systole. It forces the water out of the short, close junctions of the capillaries. The water potential is generated by the tiny solutes' tendency to flow through the walls of the capillaries.

This buildup of the solutes causes osmosis. Water moves from a high concentration (outside the vessels) to a low concentration (inside the vessels) to maintain balance. Osmotic pressure is pushing water back to the vessels. Since the blood in the capillaries is continuously circulating, the balance is never met. The equilibrium between the two powers varies at various capillary points. At the vessel's arterial point, the hydrostatic pressure is higher than the osmotic pressure, so the net flow favors water and other solutes through the tissue fluid. The osmotic pressure is stronger at the venous end, so the net flow favors the transfer of substances back to the capillary. This discrepancy is influenced by blood flow and the disparity of solutes caused by the net transport of water that favors tissue fluids.

Removal of Interstitial Fluid

The lymphatic system acts a significant role in distributing tissue fluid by preventing fluid buildup in the tissue cells. Tissue fluid flows into the surrounding lymph channels and finally enters the blood. Sometimes, tissue fluid removal does not function correctly, and there is a buildup, which is called edema. Edema is responsible for the swelling during inflammation and certain diseases where the lymphatic drainage pathways are obstructed. Capillary permeability may be improved by releasing certain cytokines, anaphylatoxins, or other mediators (including leukotrienes, prostaglandins, bradykinin, histamine, etc.) by cells after inflammation. The Starling equation determines the powers of the semipermeable membrane to determine the net flux. The explanation to the equation is known as net filtration or net flow of fluids. If the fluid is positive, it appears to leave the capillary (filtration). If negative, the fluid continues to enter the capillary (absorption). This equation has many significant physiological consequences, particularly when disease processes grossly alter one or more variables.

Capillary Dynamics: Oncotic force exerted by proteins in the blood plasma helps to draw water into the circulatory system.

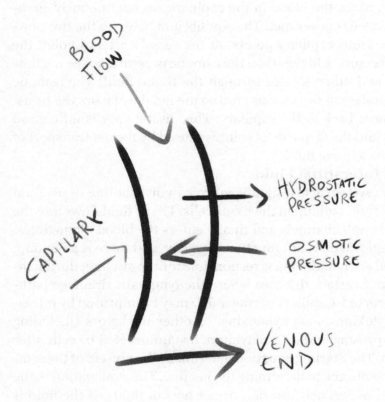

BLOOD FLOW

CAPILLARY

HYDROSTATIC PRESSURE

OSMOTIC PRESSURE

VENOUS END

Regulation of Water Intake

Water Intake

Fluid can reach the body as preformed water, ingested food, drink, and in a lesser degree as metabolic water created as a by-product of aerobic respiration and dehydration synthesis. A constant supply is required to replenish the fluids lost by normal physiological processes, such as breathing, sweating, and urination. Water produced from the biochemical metabolism of nutrients provides a large proportion of the daily water needs for certain arthropods and desert animals, but provides only a small fraction of the human intake required. In typical resting conditions, the ingestion of water by swallowed fluids is roughly 2500 ml/day. Body water homeostasis is primarily controlled by ingested fluids, which in turn depend on thirst. Thirst is the fundamental desire or impulse that drives the body to drink water.

Thirst is a feeling produced by the hypothalamus, the human body's thirst core. Thirst is an essential component of the regulation of blood volume, which is steadily controlled by homeostasis.

Hypothalamus-Mediated Thirst

The osmoreceptor is a sensory receptor that senses variations in osmotic pressure and is located predominantly in most homeothermic species' hypothalamus. Osmoreceptors track variations in plasma osmolarity (i.e., the concentration of solutes absorbed in the blood).

Since the blood's osmolarity varies (it is more or less dilute), water diffusion into and out of the osmoreceptor cells changes, cells expand as the blood plasma is more depleted and contract at a greater concentration. When osmoreceptors sense elevated plasma osmolarity (often a sign of low blood volume), they transmit messages to the hypothalamus, producing a biochemical feeling of hunger. Osmoreceptors also induce vasopressin (ADH) release, which causes events that decrease plasma osmolality to normal amounts.

Renin-Angiotensin System-Mediated Thirst

Another way of thirst is caused by angiotensin II, one of the hormones active in the renin-angiotensin mechanism. Renin-angiotensin is a complex homeostatic pathway that works with blood volume as a whole and plasma osmolarity and blood pressure. Another form of osmoreceptor is the macula densa cells found in the walls of the ascending loop of Henle of the nephron; however, it activates the juxtaglomerular apparatus (JGA) rather than the hypothalamus.

The hypothalamus is the human body's thirst center.

When the macula densa cells are activated by elevated osmolarity, the JGA releases renin into the bloodstream, which converts angiotensinogen into angiotensin I. Angiotensin I is converted to angiotensin II by ACE in the lungs. ACE is a hormone with multiple roles. Angiotensin II works on the hypothalamus to induce a sense of thirst. It also induces vasoconstriction and aldosterone release to improve the reabsorption of water in a related ADH mechanism. Note that the renin-angiotensin system, and therefore thirst, can be caused by stimuli other than increased plasma osmolarity or reduced blood volume, e.g. stimulation of the sympathetic nervous system and low blood pressure in the kidneys (lower GFR) can activate the renin-angiotensin system and increase thirst.

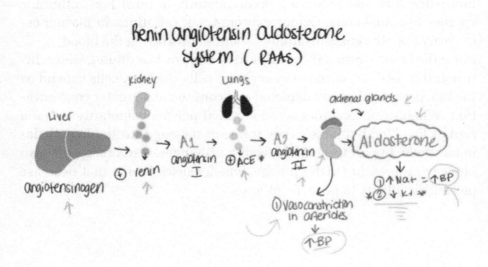

Regulation of Water Output

Water Output

Fluid will leave the body in three different ways:

1. Urine
2. Feces
3. Sweating

The main source of fluid output results from urination at approximately 1500 ml/day (approximately 1.59 qt/day) in a typical adult in a resting state. A smaller amount of fluid is lost by perspiration (part of the body's temperature regulation mechanism) and also includes the water vapor in expired air, though these fluid losses are usually smaller. The body's homeostatic regulation systems maintain a steady internal environment to regulate fluid gain and fluid loss. The hormones ADH (antidiuretic hormone, also identified as vasopressin) and aldosterone, a hormone released by the renin-angiotensin system, play a key role in this equilibrium. If the body is deficient in water, there may be an increase in these hormones' secretion, which allows the kidneys to absorb water by increased tubular reabsorption and decreased urine production. Conversely, if the fluid levels are excessive, these hormones' release is suppressed, resulting in decreased fluid accumulation in the kidneys and a corresponding rise in urinary production due to diminished fluid retention.

ADH Feedback

When blood volume is too low, plasma osmolarity can rise due to higher amounts of solutes per volume of water. Hypothalamus osmoreceptors sense elevated plasma osmolarity and activate the posterior pituitary gland to secrete ADH. ADH allows the distal convoluted tubular walls and the collecting duct to become permeable to water—this greatly increases the volume of water reabsorbed during tubular reabsorption. ADH also has a vasoconstrictive effect on the cardiovascular system, making it one of the most powerful countervailing factors during hypovolemic shock (shock from excess fluid loss or bleeding).

Aldosterone Feedback

Aldosterone is a steroid hormone (corticoid) formed at the end of the renin-angiotensin system. Low blood volume stimulates the juxtaglomerular apparatus in several ways to secrete renin. Renin cleaves angiotensin I from the liver-angiotensinogen made. Angiotensin-converting enzyme (ACE) in the lungs transforms angiotensin I to angiotensin II. Angiotensin II has different symptoms (such as increased thirst) and extracts aldosterone from the adrenal cortex. Aldosterone has a variety of effects that are involved in the control of water output. It works on mineral corticosteroid receptors in the distal convoluted tubules' epithelial cells, and collects the duct to increase the Na+/K+ ATPase pumps' expression and activate these pumps. This significantly increases sodium and water (which follows sodium osmotically through co-transport), thereby inducing potassium secretion in the urine. Aldosterone enhances the reabsorption of water; moreover, it requires an interaction of sodium and potassium that does not require ADH's reabsorption. Aldosterone can also induce a similar ion-balancing reaction in the colon and salivary glands.

Water Content in Foods

Source: National Nutrient Database for Standard Reference, Release 23

Percentage	Food Item
90–99	Nonfat milk, cantaloupe, strawberries, watermelon, lettuce, cabbage, celery, spinach, squash
80–89	Fruit juice, yogurt, apples, grapes, oranges, carrots, broccoli, pears, pineapple
70–79	Bananas, avocados, cottage cheese, ricotta cheese, baked potato, shrimp
60–69	Pasta, legumes, salmon, chicken breast
50–59	Ground beef, hot dogs, steak, feta cheese
40–49	Pizza
30–39	Cheddar cheese, bagels, bread
20–29	Pepperoni, cake, biscuits
10–19	Butter, margarine, raisins
1–9	Walnuts, dry-roasted peanuts, crackers, cereals, pretzels, peanut butter
0	Oils, sugars

Water Balance Disorders

In physiology and medicine, dehydration (hypohydration) is characterized as excessive body fluid loss. It is about extraction of water from the body. In biochemical terminology, however, this involves a deficiency of fluid within the body. Many of the biochemical consequences of dehydration are attributed to ion-concentration shifts in the said state of dehydration. Alternatively, hypovolemia can occur due to a lack of blood volume.

Dehydration

There are three forms of dehydration depending on changes in the sodium ion concentration: **Hypotonic**: primarily a loss of electrolytes, especially sodium. Hypotonic dehydration causes decreased plasma osmolality. **Hypertonic**: primarily a loss of water. Hypertonic dehydration causes increased plasma osmolality. **Isotonic:** equal reduction of water and electrolytes. Isotonic dehydration does not affect plasma osmolarity but decreases total plasma volume. Isotonic dehydration is the most common type of dehydration. There could also be more complications. In hypotonic dehydration, intravascular water transfers to extravascular space and exaggerates intravascular volume depletion due to a given sum of total body water loss.

Dehydration: Clinical Presentation

In patients with dehydration, especially infants, the following must be considered:

Intake of fluids, including volume, form (hypertonic or hypotonic), and frequency. **Urine production**, including flushing frequency (last wet diaper), presence of condensed or diluted urine, hematuria. **Method of combining baby formula:** the volume of water to powder used. **The output of stools**, frequency of stools, consistency of stools, blood or mucus in stools. **Emesis**, with frequency and volume, whether bilious or non-bilious, hematemesis

Interaction with sick people, especially other people with gastroenteritis, utilization of daycare. **Underlying conditions** such as cystic fibrosis, diabetes mellitus, hyperthyroidism, kidney disorder. **Fever. Patterns of appetite. Weight loss:** a calculation of recent weight versus weight on presentation. **Travel. Recent antibiotic use. Possible ingestions.**

Physical Examination

A complete physical examination may help to determine the patient's underlying cause of dehydration and define the severity of dehydration. The strategy of treatment is decided by a scientific evaluation of the severity of dehydration. Instead of allocating an exact percentage of dehydration, an effort should be made to put the patient, especially an infant, in one of three broad groups.

Signs and symptoms	Mild Dehydration	Moderate Dehydration	Severe Dehydration
Level of consciousness	Attentive and alert	Lethargic	Obtunded
Capillary refill*	2 s or less	2-4 s	>4 s, cool peripheries
Mucous membranes	Normal	Dry	Dry, cracked
Tears	Normal	Reduced	Absent
Heart rate	Slightly Rapid	Rapid	Very Rapid
Respiratory rate/pattern*	Normal	Increased	Increased and hyperpnea
Blood pressure	Normal	Normal, but orthostasis	Decreased
Pulse	Normal	Thready	Distant or impalpable
Skin turgor*	Normal	Slow	Tenting
Fontanelle	Normal	Depressed	Sunken
Eyes	Normal	Sunken	Very sunken
Urine output	Reduced	Oliguria	Oliguria/anuria
* Best indicators of hydration status			

Estimated Fluid Deficit

Severity	Infants (weight < 10 kg)	Children (weight >10 kg)
Mild dehydration	5% or 50 mL/kg	3% or 30 mL/kg
Moderate dehydration	10% or 100 mL/kg	6% or 60 mL/kg
Severe dehydration	15% or 150 mL/kg	9% or 90 mL/kg

Neurological complications may occur in hypotonic and hypertonic conditions. The former might lead to seizures, while the latter can progress to osmotic cerebral edema following rapid rehydration.

Treatment for Dehydration in adults

To treat mild dehydration, water consumption must be increased, while the cause of the fluid loss must be decreased or stopped entirely. Simple water restores only the amount of plasma in the blood and prevents the process of hunger until the solute levels can be refilled. Solid foods can lead to fluid loss due to vomiting and diarrhea. Mild to moderate dehydration with ORT may typically be handled very effectively. Vomiting is not necessarily a contraindication to ORT. If there is an indication of intestinal obstruction, ileus, or acute abdominal pain, intravenous rehydration is recommended. Mild to moderate dehydration with ORT may typically be handled very effectively.

WHO-UNICEF Oral Rehydration Solutions

Solution	Sodium (mEq/L)	Chloride (mEq/L)	Glucose, Anhydrous (mEq/L)	Potassium (mEq/L)	Citrate (mEq/L)	Osmolality
Basic	90	80	111	20	10	311
Decreased osmolarity	75	65	75	20	10	245

Calculate the deficit in fluids. Physical findings consistent with mild dehydration indicate a fluid deficiency of 5 percent in babies, and 3 percent in children or patients with more than 10 kg weight. Moderate dehydration happens with a fluid loss of 5-10 percent in infants, and 3-6 percent in children or in patients with more than 10 kg weight. The fluid deficit should be replaced for over 4 hours. A recorded recent weight shift remains the baseline for measuring the fluid deficit if the values are valid. Oral rehydration solution should be given very regularly in limited amounts to prevent gastric distension and reflex vomiting. Usually, 5 ml of oral rehydration solution is well tolerated per minute. The caregiver is expected to report hourly intake and output. Once the patient is rehydrated, vomiting also reduces, and higher amounts of fluids may be used. Infusion of oral rehydration solution via a nasogastric tube can be used temporarily to achieve rehydration if vomiting occurs. Intravenous fluid administration (20-30 mL/kg isotonic sodium chloride 0.9 percent solution over 1-2 h) can also be used before oral rehydration is tolerated. Replenish ongoing losses from stools and vomiting (estimate the volume and replace) in addition to replacing the calculated fluid deficit. An appropriate diet may be started as soon as the patient can tolerate oral feed.

Severe dehydration

Laboratory examination and intravenous rehydration are required. The root cause of dehydration must be determined and adequately handled. **Step 1** works on emergency response and the preservation of hemodynamic integrity. Extreme dehydration is characterized by a diagnosis of hypovolemic shock requiring immediate care. Initial treatment includes the insertion of an intravenous or intraosseous line and the quick administration of 20 mL/kg isotonic crystalloid (e.g. lactated Ringer solution, 0.9% sodium chloride). Additional fluid boluses may be expected based on the nature of the dehydration. The patient should be reassessed periodically to decide the response to therapy. When intravascular volume is replenished, both tachycardia, capillary refill, urinary output, and mental state should be restored. Suppose that improvement is not observed after 60 mL/kg of fluid administration? In that case, other etiologies of shock (e.g. cardiac, may be more evident following the preliminary fluid bolus before reaching 60 mL/kg – confirmation of a gallop rhythm on examination, rales, anaphylactic, septic) should be considered. Hemodynamic surveillance and inotropic assistance could be indicated.

Step 2 focuses on unmet shortfall substitution since phase 1, supplying maintenance fluids and replacing existing losses. Maintenance fluid specifications are equal to estimated fluid losses (urine, stool) plus insensitive fluid losses. Natural insensible fluid loss is roughly 400-500 mL/m2 of body surface area and can be exacerbated by fever and tachypnea conditions. Alternatively, the daily maintenance criteria (not including continuous pathological loss) of fluids can be approximately measured as follows:

• Body weight less than 10 kg = 100 mL/kg
• Body weight 10-20 kg = 1000 + 50 mL/kg for each kg over 10 kg
• Body weight greater than 20 kg = 1500 + 20 mL/kg for each kg above 20 kg

Severe deficiency by clinical review shows a fluid deficiency of 10-15 percent of body weight in infants and 6-9 percent of body weight in older adolescents. The fluid deficiency is applied to the normal maintenance fluid. The prescribed dosage is one-half of this amount given over 8 hours, and the rest administered over the next 16 hours. Continued casualties (e.g. emesis, diarrhea) must be immediately substituted. If the patient is isonatremic (130-150 mEq/L), the sodium deficit can usually be resolved by administering the remaining fluid deficit after step 1, plus 5 percent dextrose in 0.45-0.9 percent sodium chloride. Potassium (20 mEq/L potassium chloride) can be applied to the maintenance fluid until urine output is determined and serum potassium levels are within a reasonable range. The alternative approach to deficit treatment is quick replacement therapy. In this method, 20-40 mL/kg isotonic sodium chloride solution or lactate Ringer solution is given to a patient with severe isonatremic dehydration for 15-60 minutes. When perfusion is improved, the patient recovers and can withstand oral rehydration for the duration of the rehydration. This method is not suitable for hypernatremic or hyponatremic dehydration.

Hyponatremic dehydration

Treatment of hyponatremic dehydration is the same as that of isonatremic dehydration. Rapid volume expansion with 20 mL/kg isotonic (0.9 percent) sodium chloride solution or lactate Ringer solution can be applied and replicated before the perfusion is restored.

Severe hyponatremia (< 130 mEq/L) suggests additional sodium loss over water loss. In step 2 management, rehydration is estimated as isonatremic dehydration. The additional sodium shortfall must be measured and applied to the rehydration solution. The deficit can be estimated to restore sodium to 130 mEq/L and dispensed over 48 hours, as follows:

- Sodium deficiency = (sodium desired-sodium original) X volume of distribution X weight (kg)
- Example: sodium = 123, weight = 10 kg, assumed distribution volume 0.6; sodium deficiency = (130-123) X 0.6 X 10 kg = 42 mEq sodium

The simplified strategy is to use 5 percent dextrose in 0.9 percent sodium chloride as a replacement fluid. Sodium is closely monitored, and the level of sodium in the fluid is regulated to ensure a gradual correction (about <0.5 mEq/L/h, with a correction goal of 8 mEq/L for 24 hours). The serum sodium level must be reassessed periodically during the correction. The rapid correction of chronic hyponatremia (>2 mEq/L/h) would be consistent with central pontine myelinolysis. Rapid partial correction of symptomatic hyponatremia has still not been associated with adverse reactions. Therefore if the patient is symptomatic (seizures), a more urgent partial correction is suggested. Hypertonic (3 percent) sodium chloride solution (0.5 mEq/mL) can be used for easy partial correction of symptomatic hyponatremia. The bolus dosage of 4 mL/kg increases serum sodium by 3-4 mEq/L.

Hypernatremic dehydration

Treatment for hypernatremic dehydration is the same as for isonatremic dehydration. Rapid expansion with 20 mL/kg isotonic sodium chloride solution or lactate Ringer solution should be administered and repeated until good perfusion is established. Varied regimens can be pursued successfully to correct extreme hypernatremia (>150 mEq/L). The most important phase 2 management goal is to reestablish intravascular volume, if not done in stage 1, and correct serum sodium levels. However, this correction toward the reference range should not be more than 10 mEq/L/24h. Rapid correction of hypernatremic dehydration may have catastrophic neurological effects, including cerebral edema and death. The most prudent approach is to schedule a steady reversal of the fluid deficit over 48 hours. Rehydration fluids with 5 percent dextrose in 0.9 percent sodium chloride should be begun after sufficient intravascular volume expansion. Serum sodium levels should be measured every 2-4 hours.

If the sodium has reduced by less than 0.5 mEq/L/h, then the rehydration fluid's sodium content is decreased. This makes a gradual, regulated correction of the hypernatremic state. Hyperglycemia and hypocalcemia are also correlated with hypernatremic dehydration. Serum glucose and calcium levels should be observed closely.

Treatment of dehydration in Children

For severe dehydration, **Treat shock** if present. If able to drink, **administer oral rehydration solution** (ORS) PO while obtaining IV access. **Insert peripheral IV line** using a large-caliber catheter (22-24G in children or 18G in adults) or intraosseous needle. Administer **Ringer lactate** (RL) according to WHO Treatment Plan C, monitoring infusion rate closely:

WHO Treatment Plan C

Age	First, give 30 ml/kg over	Then, give 70 ml/kg over
Children < 1 year	1 hour	5 hours
Children ≥ 1 year and adults	30 minutes	2 ½ hours

Repeat bolus once if radial pulse remains weak or absent after the first bolus. In case of suspected severe anemia, measure hemoglobin, and treat accordingly. As soon as the patient can drink safely (often within 2 hours), provide ORS as the patient tolerates. ORS contains glucose and electrolytes, which prevent further complications. Observe for ongoing losses closely. Evaluate clinical condition and degree of dehydration at regular intervals to the continuation of appropriate treatment. *For some dehydration,* according to WHO Treatment Plan B, administering ORS equates to 75 ml/kg ORS given over 4 hours.

WHO Treatment Plan B

Age	< 4 months	4 to 11 months	12 to 23 months	2 to 4 years	5 to 14 years	≥ 15 years
Weight	< 5 kg	5 to 7.9 kg	8 to 10.9 kg	11 to 15.9 kg	16 to 29.9 kg	≥ 30 kg
Amount of ORS over 4 hours	200 to 400 ml	400 to 600 ml	600 to 800 ml	800 to 1200 ml	1200 to 2200 ml	2200 to 4000 ml

Persuade for additional age-appropriate fluid intake, including breast-feeding in young children. Give additional ORS after each loose stool (see below). Monitor ongoing losses closely. Assess clinical condition and degree of dehydration at regular intervals to ensure the continuation of appropriate treatment.

In case of *no dehydration,*

prevent dehydration: encourage age-appropriate fluid intake, including breastfeeding in young children. Administer ORS according to WHO Treatment Plan A after any loose stool.

WHO Treatment Plan A

Age	Quantity of ORS
Children < 2 years	50 to 100 ml or *10 to 20 tea-spoons*
Children 2 to 10 years	100 to 200 ml *or ½ to 1 glass*
Children over 10 years and adults	at least 250 ml or *at least 1 glass*

Hypovolemia

Hypovolemia is, in particular, a reduction in the amount of blood plasma. In comparison, hypovolemia describes the water deficit in terms of blood volume rather than the body's total water content. Intravenous fluid administration is an important therapy for correcting dehydration and hypovolemia.

Hypovolemia is a source of hypovolemic shock. Shock is a medical condition in which the body's fluids cannot circulate properly and oxygenate the human body's major organs; this causes compensatory mechanisms to activate that cause further bodily harm, as the body's metabolism is maintained longer.

In hypovolemic shock, tissue metabolism is compromised due to a loss of blood volume, making it impossible for red blood cells to enter all body tissues. It is most commonly caused by extreme vomiting, diarrhea, blood loss, or bleeding. Other types of shock with related effects include heart attacks (cardiogenic) or bacterial infections (septic).

Fluid Therapy in Special Conditions
Patients with mild to severe volume contraction, and patients with shock due to several causes are frequently admitted to medical service and the intensive care units for management. Besides, patients with pulmonary disease and patients with renal failure develop problems with fluid management. Also, patients with burns, traumatic hemorrhage, and stroke are admitted to surgical service with fluid and electrolyte problems. Therefore, a brief discussion of fluid and electrolyte therapy in these conditions is presented below.

VOLUME CONTRACTION

Elderly patients and patients from nursing homes are admitted with severe dehydration (volume depletion) because of poor oral intake and the inability to access water. These patients generally present with altered mental status, hypotension, and fever. The choice of fluid therapy is normal (0.9%) saline. Ringer's lactate can also be used if the patient has multiple electrolyte deficits. The fluids can be continued until the blood pressure, and urine output starts improving. Fever, in the absence of infection, also improves with adequate volume replacement, and the patient becomes further alert. With adequate volume replacement, all abnormal laboratory findings return to baseline or normal.

SEPTIC SHOCK

Septic shock is a condition of altered vascular permeability, fluid leakage into the extravascular space, and multiorgan involvement. Large fluid deficits (up to 10 L) are present in the septic patient. Therefore, fluid therapy is essential to improve cardiac output, blood pressure, and tissue perfusion. Isotonic saline is preferred initially to improve volume status. Fluid challenges of 1 L of saline can be given with CVP monitoring. Ringer's lactate, if indicated, can be used. Routine use of colloids is not recommended unless the patient has anemia, in which case packed RBCs are infused to raise Hb level to 9–10 g/dL. Occasionally, patients need an infusion of 25% albumin to raise serum albumin levels >2 g/dL and minimize peripheral edema. Vasopressor support is required if crystalloids alone do not improve blood pressure. Three hundred to 500 mL of colloids can also be given in 30 min. to improve hemodynamics. As mentioned above, normal saline is widely used as a volume expander in patients with septic shock. However, infusion of balanced solutions has been shown to cause fewer adverse effects, such as hyperchloremic metabolic acidosis and acute kidney injury. The cost of these balanced solutions limits their use worldwide.

HEMORRHAGIC SHOCK DUE TO GASTROINTESTINAL BLEEDING
Hemorrhagic shock can result from massive gastrointestinal bleeding. The therapeutic goals are to restore the circulating blood volume and to restore adequate Hb levels. Transfusion of packed RBCs is recommended if the Hb level is <7 g/dL. Raising the Hb level above 9–10 g/dL is not necessary. Patients with Hb levels between 7 and 10 g/dL should be evaluated for clinical instability and inadequate oxygen delivery. If the Hb level is stable, administration of crystalloids (isotonic saline) is preferred. Frequently, patients need both transfusions of packed RBCs and administration of normal saline to prevent vascular collapse.

HEMORRHAGIC SHOCK DUE TO TRAUMA
The important therapeutic goals are to improve the circulating blood volume and to restore adequate Hb levels. Crystalloid solutions are very effective in restoring intravascular volume. Therefore, crystalloid solutions are an ideal first-line treatment that should be started as soon as possible. The fluid of choice is Ringer's lactate because it can replace some of the interstitial fluid and electrolyte deficits present during hypovolemic shock. It is recommended that trauma patients receive a blood transfusion if they are not stabilized after receiving 2 L of Ringer's lactate or deteriorating following a brief stabilization. Transfusion of packed RBCs is required if the Hb level is <7 g/dL. Maintenance of Hb levels >9–10 g/ dL is not beneficial. Transfusion of FFP is indicated for coagulopathy and platelet transfusion for a platelet count <100,000/μL. Hypertonic saline (7.5%) alone or in combination with 6% dextran is also effective for trauma patients, particularly in patients with head trauma. It lowers the volume requirements and also improves survival in these patients requiring surgery.

CARDIOGENIC SHOCK

Cardiogenic shock is usually not associated with increased microvascular permeability. Therefore, the fluid requirement is not substantial. A crystalloid solution is probably the initial fluid therapy choice because the cardiogenic shock patients are not hypo-oncotic. The use of colloids can lead to changes in cardiac filling pressure, resulting in pulmonary vascular congestion. Crystalloid therapy is usually guided by pulmonary capillary wedge pressure, and cardiac output.

ADULT RESPIRATORY DISTRESS SYNDROME (ARDS)

Because of generalized vascular permeability changes, patients with ARDS demonstrate signs of decreased intravascular volume and circulatory shock, as well as pulmonary alveolar edema and hypoxemia. The management, therefore, involves restoration of intravascular volume and preservation of gas exchange. Both crystalloid and colloid therapy have been found to be effective and safe; however, crystalloid (saline) infusion may occasionally worsen pulmonary edema without impairing gas exchange. Therefore, colloid rather than crystalloid infusion is suggested. Furthermore, colloids are more potent volume-expanders than crystalloids and produce greater cardiac output and systemic oxygen delivery. Despite these beneficial effects, crystalloids are generally recommended in most patients with ARDS unless the patients are anemic and have hypoalbuminemia, in which case colloids are the choice of fluid resuscitation. The major goal of fluid therapy in ARDS is to minimize the increases in pulmonary hydrostatic pressure. For this purpose, frequent pulmonary capillary wedge pressure, or CVP and radiographic measurements, and clinical evaluation for pulmonary edema are essential.

Phases of Fluid Therapy in Critically Ill Patients

Fluid therapy is an early intervention in the management of acutely ill patients. The selection of resuscitation fluid should be based on the patient's clinical context. The need for fluid therapy in critically ill patients is not static, but varies depending on the hemodynamic status. Therefore, a conceptual model for fluid management has been proposed. This model includes four phases: (1) rescue or salvage, (2) optimization, (3) stabilization, and (4) de-escalation.

- The rescue phase is characterized by life-threatening shock (hypotension and poor organ perfusion), which requires rapid fluid bolus therapy.
- The optimization phase is less life-threatening and requires fluid boluses of 250–500 mL in 15–20 min. to restore cardiac output and organ perfusion.
- During the stabilization phase, fluid management aims to maintain adequate intravascular volume (maintenance of fluid balance).
- The de-escalation phase is characterized by recovery measures, including weaning from the ventilator and vasoactive support, and volume overload treatment by appropriate measures.
-

It should be remembered that these processes are not mutually exclusive, but are interrelated.

Intravenous Fluids

This topic reviews various fluids available for intravenous (IV) administration. IV fluids can be classified into two categories: Varied regimens can be pursued successfully to correct extreme hypernatremia (>150 mEq/L). The most critical objective in phase 2 management is to recover intravascular volume if not reached at stage 1, and return serum sodium levels to the reference range by no more than 10 mEq/L/24h. crystalloids and colloids. Crystalloids are solutions that contain water, electrolytes, and/or glucose, whereas colloids are mainly albumin and blood products. IV solutions can be categorized as isotonic, hypotonic, or hypertonic. In general, isotonic solutions are often used to treat extracellular fluid (ECF) loss, hypotonic solutions to restore ECF and intracellular fluid (ICF) depletion, and hypertonic solutions to correct symptomatic hyponatremia. Hypertonic saline is often used in emergency settings, as it lowers intracranial pressure in patients with head injuries and patients with burns. It is important to know the formulation of the widely used crystalloids and colloids so that we can understand their indications.

Crystalloids
Dextrose Water
- Dextrose water is available as a 2.5, 5, 10, and 50 percent (comprising 25, 50, 100, and 500 g dextrose in 1 L of water, correspondingly).
- Dextrose is metabolized into water and CO_2, and the water is dispersed between ECF and ICF compartments.
- The most widely used clinical management approach is 5 percent dextrose in water, which is generally abbreviated as D5W. This solution is 170 kcal/L. Clearwater induces hemolysis when administered intravenously; thus, D5W is used to supply pure water.

Sodium Chloride (NaCl) containing Liquids

- NaCl is available in concentrations of 0.225, 0.45, 0.9, 3 and 5 percent (comprising 38.5, 77.154, 513 and 1250 mEq of Na+ and equivalent Cl– in 1 L) solutions.
- 0.9 percent NaCl solution is generally referred to as normal or isotonic saline, while 0.225 and 0.45 percent NaCl are referred to as hypotonic fluids. For example, 1 L of 0.45 percent of saline contains 500 mL of isotonic solution and 500 mL of free water. As a result, 0.45 percent NaCl solution offers more free water than 0.9 percent NaCl solution.
- Because insensible losses are poor in electrolytes, hypotonic solutions are commonly known to be true maintenance fluids.
- In common, 3, 5, and 7.5% NaCl are called hypertonic solutions.
- Normal saline is the most commonly used crystalloid worldwide.
- Infusion of 1 L normal saline to a healthy individual expands intravascular volume by 20%. Moreover, the infused volume remains in the vascular space for approximately 30 min.
- Recent studies have shown that infusion of solutions containing high Cl– to critically ill patients has caused some adverse effects, such as hyperchloremic metabolic acidosis and acute kidney injury.
- Balanced electrolyte solutions with low Cl– concentration, on the other hand, caused fewer adverse effects compared to normal saline.

Dextrose in Saline
Dextrose saline is available as D5 0.225, D5 0.45, and D5 0.9 percent solutions. These fluids supply Na+, Cl–, free water, and 170 kcal/L.

Balanced Electrolyte Solutions

- There are several "balanced" electrolyte solutions such as Ringer's lactate (also called lactated Ringer's), Ringer's acetate, normosol R, Plasma-Lyte 148, and isolyte S are available for use; however, Ringer's lactate is the most frequently used solution in fluid therapy because of its consideration as being a *physiologic saline.*

- Both lactate and acetate are converted to HCO3 – in the liver. Also, both are vasodilators.
- Ringer's lactate contains fewer Na+ than normal saline, and it is approximately 10% less effective as a volume expander than normal saline. Also, it is not a recommended
- solution in patients with renal failure because of K+.

Colloids

Albumin

Albumin is the most frequently used colloid in clinical practice. It is extracted from human plasma and is available as 5 or 25% in normal saline. The primary role of albumin is to maintain intravascular on-cotic pressure. Albumin stays in
the intravascular compartment for at least 16 h before it diffuses into the interstitial space.
The practice of using albumin as a volume expander should be individualized.

Indications for albumin

1. To expand plasma volume when crystalloids have failed to correct acutely diminished intravascular volume
2. To treat severe edematous patients with nephrotic syndrome resistant to potent diuretic therapy
3. To prevent hemodynamic instability and acute kidney injury following large volume (>5 L) paracentesis
4. To prevent renal impairment and mortality in patients with spontaneous bacterial peritonitis
5. To treat cirrhotic patients with hypoalbuminemia and hypovolemia
6. To treat hepatorenal syndrome with other agents (midodrine, octreotide)
7. To replace plasma volume during plasmapheresis
8. *Do not* use to treat hypoalbuminemia due to malnutrition unless the patient has protein-losing enteropathy

9. *Do not* use routinely in critically ill patients with hypovolemia, burns, or hypoalbuminemia because albumin administration does not *reduce* mortality.

Goals of Fluid Therapy

• To normalize hemodynamic and electrolyte abnormalities
• To maintain daily requirements of fluids and electrolytes
• To replace previous fluid and electrolyte losses
• To replace ongoing fluid and electrolyte losses
• To provide nutrition
• To provide a source for IV drug administration.

Choice of fluid

The choice of fluid therapy depends largely on the clinical situation. Crystalloids are usually preferred to colloids in fluid therapy except in certain situations. Fluid therapy is not without complications. Some of the complications include fluid overload, pulmonary edema; electrolyte disturbances such as hyponatremia with hypotonic solutions and hypernatremia with hypertonic solutions, IV catheter-associated infections, and phlebitis. Dangerous hyperkalemia may develop with K+-containing solutions, particularly in patients with renal failure. Also, hyperchloremic metabolic acidosis (dilutional acidosis) and acute kidney injury may develop with large volumes of normal saline.

Edema and volume-overload

Edema is an aggregation of fluid in the interstitial space that arises as capillary filtration reaches the thresholds of lymphatic drainage, causing visible clinical signs and symptoms. The rapid progression of generalized pitting edema associated with systemic disease demands timely diagnosis and treatment. Prolonged accumulation of edema in one or both lower extremities often suggests a venous insufficiency, particularly in the existence of dependent edema and hemosiderin deposition. Skin treatment is essential to the prevention of skin breakdown and venous ulcers. Eczematous (static) dermatitis should be treated with emollients and topical steroid creams. Patients with deep venous thrombosis should wear compression stockings to avoid post-thrombotic syndrome. If the clinical suspicion of deep venous thrombosis remains elevated, after negative findings on duplex ultrasonography have been observed, further examination can require magnetic resonance venography to rule out pelvic or thigh proximal venous thrombosis or compression. Obstructive sleep apnea can induce bilateral leg edema even in the absence of pulmonary hypertension. Brawny, non-pitting edema characterizes lymphedema, which can be found in one or both lower extremities. Possible indirect causes of lymphedema include tumor, fracture, recent pelvic surgery, inguinal lymphadenectomy, and prior radiation therapy. In these situations, the use of pneumatic compression devices or compression stockings can be beneficial.

Mechanism of edema in different conditions
SYSTEMIC
- Allergic reaction, urticaria, and angioedema
- Enhanced capillary permeability
- Cardiac disease (Increased capillary permeability due to systemic venous hypertension; increased plasma volume)
- Hepatic disease (Increased capillary permeability due to systemic venous hypertension; lowered oncotic plasma pressure due to reduced protein synthesis)
- Malabsorption/protein-calorie malnutrition
Decreased protein synthesis associated with decreased plasma oncotic pressure

- Obstructive sleep apnea (OSA), Pulmonary hypertension leading to elevated hydrostatic capillary pressure
- Pregnancy and premenstrual edema
- Increased plasma volume
- Renal disease, Increased plasma volume; reduced plasma oncotic pressure due to protein loss.

LOCALIZED
- *Cellulitis* (Enhanced capillary permeability)
- *Chronic venous insufficiency* (Raised capillary permeability caused by local venous hypertension)
- *Compartment syndrome* (Increased capillary permeability due to local venous hypertension)
- *Complex regional pain syndrome type 1* (also known as reflex sympathetic dystrophy)
- *Deep venous thrombosis* (Enhanced capillary permeability)
- *Iliac vein obstruction* (Enhanced capillary permeability initiated by regional venous hypertension)
- *Lipedema* (Collection of fluid in adipose tissue)
- *Lymphedema* (Lymphatic obstruction)
- *May-Thurner syndrome* (Compression of left iliac vein by a right iliac artery)
- *Enhanced capillary permeability* (Caused by local venous hypertension due to compression).

Common Causes for Localized Edema

UNILATERAL PREDOMINANCE
Chronic venous insufficiency
- Onset: chronic; begins in middle to older age
- Site: lower extremities; bilateral distribution in late stages
- Clinical findings: soft, pitting edema with reddish-hued skin; a predilection for medial ankle/calf
- Associated Clinical findings: venous ulcerations over medial malleolus; weeping erosions
- Diagnosis: duplex ultrasonography, ankle-brachial index to evaluate for arterial insufficiency

- Treatment: Compression stockings, Pneumatic compression device if stockings are contraindicated
- Horse-chestnut seed extract
- Skincare (e.g. emollients and topical steroids).

Deep venous thrombosis (DVT)
- Onset: acute
- Site: upper or lower extremities
- Clinical findings: pitting edema with tenderness, with or without erythema; positive Homans sign
- Diagnosis: duplex ultrasonography, d-dimer assay, magnetic resonance venography to exclude pelvic or thigh DVT (where clinical suspicion is high) or external venous compression (May-Thurner syndrome in patients with unexplained left-sided DVT). Also, consider hypercoagulability workup
- Treatment: Compression stockings to prevent the post-thrombotic syndrome, anticoagulation therapy, thrombolysis in selected patients.

Lymphedema
- Onset: chronic; insidious; often resulting in lymphatic obstruction from trauma or surgery
- Location: upper or lower limbs; bilateral in 30% of individuals.
- Early: dough-like skin; pitting
- Late: thickened, verrucous, fibrotic, hyperkeratotic skin
- Associated findings: inability to tent skin over the second digit, swelling of the dorsum of the foot with squared-off digits, painless heaviness in extremity
- Clinical diagnosis
- Lymphoscintigraphy
- T1-weighted magnetic resonance lymphangiography
- Complex decongestive physiotherapy
- Compression stockings with adjuvant pneumatic compression devices
- Skincare
- Surgery is limited to individual cases.

Complex regional pain syndrome type 1, or Reflex sympathetic dystrophy
- Onset: Late/ chronic; following trauma or another inciting event
- Site: upper or lower extremities; contralateral limb at risk regardless of trauma
- Soft tissue edema distal to the affected limb
- Associated clinical findings: (early) warm, sensitive skin with diaphoresis; (late) thin, shiny skin with atrophic changes
- Patients: history along with examination is important for diagnosis
- Radiography
- Three-phase bone scintigraphy
- Magnetic resonance imaging
- Treatment: topical dimethyl sulfoxide solution, systemic steroids, physical therapy, tricyclic antidepressants, calcium channel blockers.

BILATERAL PREDOMINANCE
Lipedema
- Onset: chronic; begins around or after puberty
- Site: predominantly lower extremities; involves thighs, legs, buttocks; spares feet, ankles, and upper torso
- Non-pitting edema; increased distribution of soft, adipose tissue
- Associated clinical findings: medial thigh and tibial tenderness; fat pad anterior to lateral malleoli
- Diagnosis is clinical
- No effective treatment
- Weight loss does not improve edema.

Medication-induced edema
- Onset: weeks after the start of medication; resolves within days of stopping the offending medication
- Location: lower extremities
- Soft, pitting edema
- Clinical history suggesting recent initiation of the offending medication

- Cessation of medication.

Obstructive sleep apnea
- Onset: chronic
- Site: lower extremities
- Mild, pitting edema
- Associated clinical findings: daytime fatigue, snoring, and obesity
- Suggestive clinical history is very much important for diagnosis
- Diagnostic tests: polysomnography, echocardiography, and positive pressure ventilation
- Treatment: pulmonary hypertension should be treated if suggested on echocardiography.

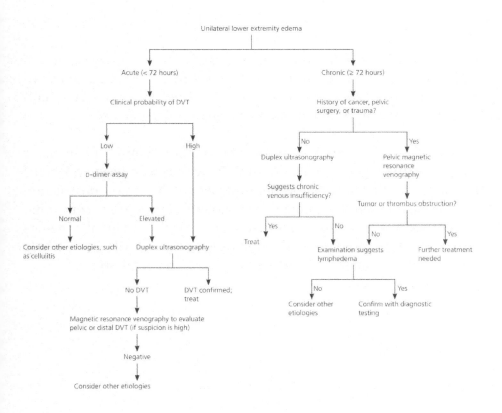

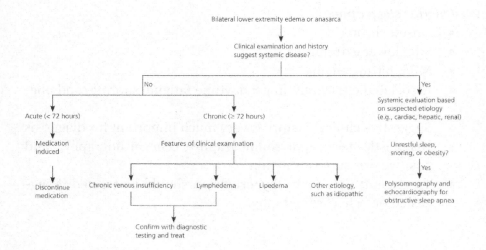

Dependent edema induced by venous insufficiency is expected to decrease with elevation and worsen with lowering the limb. Edema associated with decreased oncotic pressure (e.g. malabsorption, liver failure, nephrotic syndrome) may not change with dependence.

Unilateral swelling due to compression or compromise of venous or lymphatic drainage may result from DVT, venous insufficiency, venous tumor obstruction (e.g. iliac tumor obstruction), lymphatic obstruction (e.g. pelvic tumor or lymphoma), or lymphatic damage (e.g. congenital vs. secondary from a tumor, radiation, or filariasis). Bilateral or generalized swelling indicates a systemic origin, such as CHF (especially right-sided), pulmonary hypertension, chronic renal failure.

Assessment of Edema

History
The history should include the edema's timing, whether it changes with position, and if it is unilateral or bilateral; medication history, and an assessment for systemic diseases. Acute swelling of a limb over less than 72 hours is more characteristic of deep venous thrombosis (DVT), ruptured popliteal cyst, cellulitis, acute compartment syndrome from trauma, or recent initiation of calcium channel blockers. Prolonged accumulation of more generalized edema is attributed to the onset or exacerbation of chronic systemic diseases: for instance, congestive heart failure (CHF), kidney disease, or hepatic disease.

Medications Commonly Associated with Edema
Edema can be an adverse effect of some drugs. The process also entails the retention of salt and water with elevated capillary hydrostatic pressure. Diuretic use can induce volume depletion and reflex activation of the renin-angiotensin system.

CLASS	SPECIFIC MEDICATIONS
Antidepressants	Monoamine oxidase inhibitors, trazodone
Antihypertensives	Calcium channel blockers, Beta-adrenergic blockers, clonidine (Catapres), hydralazine, minoxidil, methyldopa
Antivirals	Acyclovir (Zovirax)
Chemotherapeutics	Cyclophosphamide (Sandimmune), cytosine arabinoside, cyclosporine, mithramycin
Cytokines	Granulocyte-macrophage colony-stimulating factor, Granulocyte colony-stimulating factor, interleukin-4 interferon alfa, interleukin-2
Hormones	Androgen, testosterone, corticosteroids, estrogen, progesterone
Nonsteroidal anti-inflammatory drugs	Celecoxib (Celebrex), ibuprofen

History should also contain concerns about heart, lung, thyroid, or hepatic disorder. Graves' disease can lead to pretibial myxedema, while hypothyroidism can cause generalized myxedema. While known to be a diagnosis of exclusion, obstructive sleep apnea has been shown to cause edema. One research tested the apnea-hypopnea index in patients with obstructive sleep apnea and showed that the body mass index and the existence of hypertension and diabetes mellitus were both balanced for age.

PHYSICAL EXAMINATION

Physical testing should be performed for structural causes of edema, such as heart dysfunction (e.g. jugular venous distention, crackles), renal ailment (e.g. oliguria, proteinuria), hepatic disease (e.g. jaundice, asterixis, ascites) or thyroid disease (e.g. exophthalmos, weight-loss tremor). Edema can also be checked for pitting, tenderness, and changes in the skin. Pitting defines the indentation that persists in the edematous region after pressure is applied. This happens because the interstitial space fluid has a low protein content associated with reduced plasma oncotic pressure, and disorders induced by elevated capillary pressure (e.g. DVT, CHF, iliac vein compression). The physician should identify the location, duration, and severity of the pitting to evaluate the treatment response. The lower extremity inspection should focus on the medial malleolus, the bone part of the tibia, and the dorsum of the foot. Pitting edema may also occur in the early stages of lymphedema due to the flow of protein-rich fluid into the interstitium; thus, its involvement does not preclude the diagnosis of lymphedema. Tenderness on palpation over the edematous area is consistent with DVT and complex regional type 1 pain syndrome (i.e. reflex sympathetic dystrophy). Conversely, lymphedema usually does not cause pain with palpation.

Changes in skin temperature, color, and texture give clues as to the source of the edema. For example, acute DVT and cellulitis can cause increased warmth in the affected region. Owing to hemosiderin, chronic venous insufficiency is frequently associated with brownish, reddish skin and usually includes the medial malleolus. As venous insufficiency progresses, lipodermatosclerosis, which is associated with marked sclerotic and hyperpigmented tissue and characterized by fibrosis and hemosiderin deposition, can lead to venous ulcers over the medial malleolus. These ulcers will lead to intense, weeping erosions. Myxedema from hypothyroidism has generalized rough, thick skin with non-pitting periorbital edema and yellow to orange skin discoloration over the knees, palms, elbows, and soles. Graves' disease may cause localized pretibial myxedema. The skin can look shiny with atrophic changes in the late stages of complex regional pain syndrome. The skin has a doughy texture in the early stages of lymphedema. At the same time, it becomes fibrotic, thickened, and verrucous in the later stages. Examination of the feet is crucial in lower extremity edema. In patients with lymphedema, there is an incapability to tent the skin of the dorsum of the second toe when applying a pincer grasp (Kaposi-Stemmer sign). In patients with lipedema, a pathological buildup of adipose tissue in the extremities, the legs are usually spared, while the ankles also have conspicuous malleolar fat pads. Lipedema can also involve the upper extremities.

DIAGNOSTIC TESTING
Recommendations for medical tests are listed below. The following laboratory procedures are useful for the detection of systemic causes of edema: brain natriuretic peptide measurement (for CHF), creatinine test and urinalysis (for kidney disease), and hepatic enzyme and albumin measurement (for hepatic disease). In patients with acute onset of unilateral upper or lower extremity swelling, a dimer enzyme-linked immunosorbent assay can exclude DVT in low-risk patients. However, this test has poor accuracy, and in the absence of thrombosis, d-dimer concentrations can be increased.

ULTRASONOGRAPHY
Venous ultrasonography is the mode of imaging of choice for the assessment of suspected DVT. Ultrasound compression, with or without Doppler waveform analysis, has a good sensitivity (95%) and specificity (96%) for proximal thrombosis, but the sensitivity is lower for calf veins (73 percent). Duplex ultrasonography may also be used to confirm the diagnosis of chronic venous insufficiency.

LYMPHOSCINTIGRAPHY
Ultrasonic lymphatic flow cannot be detected. Indirect radionuclide lymphoscintigraphy, which shows no filling or delayed filling of lymphatic channels, is, therefore, the method of choice for assessing lymphedema when the diagnosis cannot be made clinically.

MAGNETIC RESONANCE IMAGING
Patients with unilateral lower extremity edema, that does not show proximal thrombosis with duplex ultrasonography, may need further imaging to diagnose the cause of edema if the clinical presumption of DVT remains large. Magnetic resonance angiography for lower extremity venography and pelvis can be used to assess intestinal or extrinsic pelvic or thigh DVT. The left iliac vein's compression by the right iliac artery (May-Thurner syndrome) should be suspected in women between 18 and 30 who present with edema of the left lower extremity. Magnetic resonance imaging may aid in diagnosing musculoskeletal ailments, such as a gastrocnemius tear or popliteal cyst. T1-weighted magnetic resonance lymphangiography may be used to visualize the lymphatic system when lymphedema is suspected directly.

OTHER STUDIES
Echocardiography for pulmonary arterial pressure assessment is recommended for patients with obstructive sleep apnea and edema. Pulmonary hypertension is thought to be the cause of edema associated with obstructive sleep apnea.

Management of Edema

Edema treatment should be directed by underlying etiology, which typically involves chronic venous insufficiency, lymphedema, DVT, and edema-induced drugs.

CHRONIC VENOUS INSUFFICIENCY

Diuretic therapy should be avoided in patients with chronic venous insufficiency unless a comorbid condition requires it (e.g. CHF). Mechanical treatments, including leg-raising and compression straps of 20 to 30 mm Hg for moderate edema, and 30to 40 mm Hg for extreme edema exacerbated by ulceration, are advised. Compression therapy is avoided in patients with peripheral artery disease. The ankle-brachial index measurement should be considered in patients with risk factors for peripheral arterial disease before recommending compression therapy. No definite evidence exists for the use of pneumatic compression devices in individuals with chronic venous insufficiency. However, these devices should be considered in patients for whom compression stockings are contraindicated. Local skin and wound care for venous ulcers is essential for the prevention of secondary cellulitis and dermatitis. Eczematous (static) dermatitis, characterized by dry, swollen, scaling skin overlying superficial varicose veins, often occurs in patients with chronic venous insufficiency. Treatment includes daily emollient hydration and short courses of topical steroid creams for severely inflamed skin.

LYMPHEDEMA

The mainstay in lymphedema treatment includes complex decongestive physiotherapy, comprising of manual lymphatic massage and multilayer bandages. The initial aim is to enhance fluid resorption before a full therapeutic result is attained. The maintenance process of the procedure involves compression stockings of 30 to 40 mm Hg. Pneumatic compression devices have been shown to supplement standard therapies. Surgical or bypass procedures are confined to severe refractory cases. Diuretics have no part in the management of lymphedema.

DEEP VENOUS THROMBOSIS

Acute thrombotic cases are treated with anticoagulation therapy (un-fractionated or low-molecular-weight heparin or warfarin [Coumadin]) to prevent the progression of a clot or the development of the post-thrombotic syndrome. A post thrombotic syndrome is characterized by chronic swelling of the leg, pain, cramping, and skin changes, like tel-angiectasia, arising in 20% to 50% of cases within five years of a throm-botic case. In addition to anticoagulation, compression stockings after DVT can be used to avoid post-thrombotic syndrome.

MEDICATION-INDUCED EDEMA

Where appropriate, the offending drug should be stopped in patients with known edema-induced drugs. In patients undergoing calcium-channel blockers to treat hypertension, the use of angiotensin-convert-ing enzyme inhibitor may be more effective than angiotensin-receptor blocker therapy in reducing calcium-channel blocker–induced periph-eral edema.

TREATMENT FOR OTHER CAUSES:

There is no treatment for lipedema. This disease is not affected by weight loss. Complex regional pain syndrome is treated by physiother-apy paired with systemic steroids and tricyclic antidepressants. Ob-structive sleep apnea is treated by positive ventilation pressure. Treat-ment of edema is by diuretic use.

Clinical Uses of Diuretics

Diuretics' primary action is to increase Na+ and water excretion in pa-tients with edema of variable causes. Diuretics are also used to treat hypertension and other non-edematous conditions.

Disease condition	Diuretics commonly used	Mechanism/effect
Generalized edema states		
Congestive heart failure	Furosemide metolazone Spironolactone or both	↑ Excretion of Na+ and water to reduce edema
Liver cirrhosis with ascites	Spironolactone, Furosemide or both	↑ Excretion of Na+ and water prevention of hypokalemia ↓ Edema
Nephrotic syndrome	Furosemide, amiloride	↑ Excretion of Na+ and water ↓ Edema
Idiopathic edema	Hydrochlorothiazide furosemide	↓ Edema by promoting Na+ and H2O Excretion
Localized edema		
Pulmonary edema	Furosemide and bumetanide	↓ Pulmonary congestion by removing Na+and water
Cerebral edema	Mannitol	↓ Intracranial pressure
Nonedematous states		
Acute kidney injury	Furosemide and mannitol	Improve urine flow and convert oliguric (< 400 mL urine) to non-oliguric (> 400 mL urine) failure
Chronic kidney disease (GFR < 60 mL/min)	Furosemide and metolazone	↑ Excretion of Na+ and water Thiazides other than metolazone do not work at GFR < 30 mL/min
Hypertension	Thiazides	↓ Plasma volume and cardiac output
Renal calcium stones	Hydrochlorothiazide	↓ Ca2+ excretion
Nephrogenic diabetes insipidus	Hydrochlorothiazide	↓ Plasma volume and polyuria
Acute hypercalcemia	Furosemide	↓ Ca2+ absorption in the thick ascending limb and promotes calciuria
Glaucoma	Acetazolamide	↓ HCO3− and Na+ transport and ↓ aqueous humor formation

Complications of diuretic use

Chronic use of diuretics causes several complications, which can be considered under three categories:

Fluid electrolyte and acid-base disorders
Extracellular fluid volume depletion
Hyponatremia (mostly thiazide diuretics)
Hypokalemia
Hyperkalemia (K+-sparing diuretics)
Hypocalcemia and hypercalciuria (loop diuretics)
Hypercalcemia (thiazide diuretics)
Hypomagnesemia (thiazide and loop diuretics)
Hypophosphatemia (all except K+-sparing diuretics)
Metabolic acidosis (Acetazolamide and K+-sparing diuretics)
Metabolic alkalosis (thiazide and loop diuretics)
Metabolic disorders
Hyperuricemia (thiazides cause both hyper- and hypouricemia)
Hyperglycemia (thiazides and loop diuretics)
Hyperlipidemia (thiazide and loop diuretics)
Gynecomastia (mostly spironolactone)
Sexual dysfunction (mostly spironolactone)
Toxicities
Hypersensitivity reactions
Deafness
Pancreatitis
Renal calculi

Acetazolamide
"**ACID**" azolamide causes **ACID**osis.
Loop diuretics
ADVERSE EFFECTS
Loops **L**ose **Ca2+**.
Ototoxicity, **H**ypokalemia, **H**ypomagnesemia, **D**ehydration, **A**llergy (sulfa), metabolic **A**lkalosis, **N**ephritis (interstitial), **G**out.
OHH DAANG!
Loop earrings hurt your **ears**.
Thiazide diuretics
ADVERSE EFFECTS
Hypokalemic metabolic alkalosis, hyponatremia, hyper**G**lycemia, hyper**L**ipidemia, hyper**U**ricemia, hyper**C**alcemia. Sulfa allergy.
"Hyper**GLUC**"
Potassium-sparing diuretics
Spironolactone, **E**plerenone, **A**miloride, **T**riamterene.
"Ta**K**e a **SEAT**"
Angiotensin-converting enzyme inhibitors
ADVERSE EFFECTS:
Cough, **A**ngioedema, **T**eratogen (fetal renal malformations), increased **C**reatinine, **H**yperkalemia and **H**yp**o**tension
"Captopril's **CATCHH**".

Chapter 3
Serum Sodium

Sodium (Na+) is the most abundant cation present in extracellular fluid, and together with corresponding chloride and bicarbonate anions, it accounts for 92% of serum osmolality. Sodium plays a key role in maintaining homeostasis in various ways, including maintaining the extracellular fluid's osmotic pressure, controlling renal retention and excretion in water, retaining acid-base balance, managing potassium and chloride levels, triggering neuromuscular reactions, and maintaining systemic blood pressure.

Normal values:

Age	Conventional Units	SI Units (Conversion Factor X1)
Newborn	133–146 mEq/L	133–146 mmol/L
Infant	133–144 mEq/L	133–144 mmol/L
Child	135–145 mEq/L	135–145 mmol/L
Adult	135–145 mEq/L	135–145 mmol/L

Sodium imbalance:

- Hypernatremia (high sodium level) occurs when there is excessive water loss or excessive sodium retention. Hypernatremia is defined as a serum sodium level of more than 145 mmol/L. Severe symptoms only occur when levels are above 160 mmol/L.

- Hyponatremia (low sodium level) occurs when sodium retention or absorption becomes insufficient. It is defined as a sodium concentration of less than 135 mmol/L (135 mEq/L), with severe hyponatremia below 120 mEq/L.

Hyponatremia

In normal persons, hyponatremia does not develop unless water intake is greater than renal excretion. A defect in water excretion is due to high circulating levels of antidiuretic hormone (ADH). With the retention of water, hyponatremic patients are unable to lower their urine osmolality <100 mOsm/kg H2O. Hyponatremia occurs due to elevated secretion and ADH activity and the kidneys' failure to dilute urine as much as possible due to decreased water excretion.

Causes of Hyponatremia
Remember "**NO Na+**"
Na+ excretion increased with renal problems, NG suction (GI system rich in sodium), vomiting, diuretics, sweating, diarrhea, decreased secretion of aldosterone (diabetes insipidus) (wasting sodium)
Overload of fluid with congestive heart failure, hypotonic fluids infusions, renal failure (dilutes sodium)
Na+ intake low through low salt diets, or nothing by mouth
Antidiuretic hormone over-secreted **SIADH (Syndrome of Inappropriate AntiDiuretic Hormone secretion... remember, retains water in the body and this dilutes sodium)

Specific Causes of Hyponatremia
It is not easily possible to discuss every cause of hypotonic hyponatremia. However, it is important to concentrate on those disorders that are also correlated with hyponatremia.

Syndrome of Inappropriate Antidiuretic Hormone Secretion

SIADH is a disease of exclusion. Syndrome of inappropriate antidiuretic hormone (SIADH) secretion is a common cause of hyponatremia in admitted children. Typically caused by central nervous system (CNS) diseases, lung disorders, malignancies, and medications. Some drugs may stimulate the secretion, whereas other drugs may potentiate the action of ADH. Clinically, edema is absent, and blood pressure is normal.

SIADH causes
Mnemonic: SIADH
1. **S**urgery
2. **I**ntracranial – Infection, Head injury, CVA
3. **A**lveolar – Carcinoma, Pus
4. **D**rugs – Opiates, Antiepileptics, Cytotoxics, Anti-psychotics
5. **H**ormonal – Hypothyroid, Low corticosteroid level

Or

Hyponatremia causes
Adding **S**id's **H**air **D**ye **C**reates **S**eriously **L**ow **V**olume
• **A**ddison's disease
• **S**IADH
• **H**ypothyroid
• **D**iuretics (especially thiazides)
• **C**arbamazepine
• **S**SRIs
• **L**ow **V**olume – postural drop in BP

The diagnostic criteria of SIADH:

- Hypotonic hyponatremia when plasma osmolality < 270 mOsm/kg H2O
- Inappropriate urinary absorption (>100 mOsm/kg H2O) or failure to dilute urinary osmolality below 100 mOsm/kg H2O
- Urinary Na+ >30 mEq/L for daily diet
- Euvolemia
- Absence of thyroid, adrenal, liver, heart, and kidney disease.

Serum ADH levels are usually elevated in many patients due to a defect in osmoregulation.

SIADH diagnostic criteria
Mnemonic: SOD-IUM/S
1. Serum **O**smolality **D**ecreased (<275 mOsm/kg)
2. Increased **U**rine **M**olality/osmolality (>100 mOsm/kg)
Increased Urine **S**odium/Na+ (>40 Meq/L)
3. Others:
• Euvolemic (Normal skin turgor, Blood pressure within normal range)
• Absence of other causes of hyponatremia (adrenal insufficiency, hypothyroidism, cardiac failure, pituitary insufficiency, renal disease with salt wastage, hepatic disease, diuretics)
• Correction of hyponatremia with fluid restriction

Cerebral Salt Wasting or Renal Salt Wasting Syndrome

Cerebral salt wasting (CSW) is comparable to SIADH in many ways, except for hemodynamic status and management. Like SIADH, CSW is associated with CNS disease. CSW was originally identified in patients with subarachnoid hemorrhage, but this correlation was not reported in a recent review. Subsequently, it was documented in patients with tuberculosis and other infections.

Cerebral Salt Wasting Syndrome (CSWS) Causes
Mnemonic: CSWS
1. **C**ranial trauma and neoplasm
2. **S**AH (Subarachnoid hemorrhage)
3. '**W**orms', i.e., infection (meningitis, encephalitis)
4. **S**urgery

Biochemical marker	SIADH	CSWS
Intravascular volume status	Normal to high	Low
Serum sodium	Low	Low
Urinary sodium level	High	Very high
Vasopressin level	High	Low
Urine output	Normal or low	High
Serum uric acid level	Low	Low
Initial fractional excretion of urate	High	High
Fractional excretion of urate after correction of hyponatremia	Normal	High
Urinary osmolality	High	High
Serum osmolality	Low	Low
Blood urea nitrogen/creatinine level	Low to normal	High
Serum potassium level	Normal	Normal to high
Central venous pressure	Normal to high	Low
Pulmonary capillary wedge pressure	Normal to high	Low
Brain natriuretic peptide level	Normal	High
Treatment	Water restriction	Fluids and/or mineralocorticoid

CSWS = Cerebral salt wasting syndrome; SIADH = Syndrome of inappropriate antidiuretic hormone

Nephrogenic Syndrome of Inappropriate Antidiuresis

Nephrogenic Syndrome of Inappropriate Antidiuresis (NSIAD) is identical to SIADH but is rare. Unlike SIADH, NSIAD patients have undetectable or exceedingly low levels of ADH. NSIAD is a gain-of-function mutation of the V2-receptor vasopressin. Treatment is a restriction of fluid, urea, and vaptans.

Reset Osmotat

It is a variant of SIADH because of euvolemia and hyponatremia. Usually, serum Na+ levels remain between 125 and 130 mEq/L despite variable salt and water intake. Patients with reset osmostat are usually asymptomatic, and their kidneys have normal function. Pathogenesis is unclear; however, ADH secretion occurs at low plasma osmolality (<280 mOsm/kg H2O). Patients with alcoholism, malnutrition, spinal cord injury, tuberculosis, and cerebral palsy are prone to develop reset osmostat. Also, a reset osmostat is seen in normal pregnancy. Long-term use of DDAVP has been implicated in reset osmostat. Distinguishing features from classic SIADH are:

(1) preservation of both diluting and concentrating capabilities

(2) normal Uric acid

(3) failure of fluid restriction to improve hyponatremia.

Thiazide Diuretics

Hyponatremia is a well-known side effect of thiazide diuretics. The major reason for hyponatremia is the inability to dilute urine osmolality below 100 mOsm/kg H2O because of impaired water excretion. Urine concentrating ability is preserved. Other mechanisms of hyponatremia include:

(1) volume contraction,

(2) early diuretic-induced inactivation of the tubuloglomerular feedback system;

(3) decreased glomerular filtration rate (GFR) due to the previous two mechanisms;

(4) increased ADH release and increased resorption of water;

(5) the relative drop in vasodilatory prostaglandin synthesis in elderly subjects with non-adverse ADH activity.

• Diuretic-induced hypokalemia can further intensify hyponatremia by a transcellular cation exchange in which K+ moves out of the cell to enhance hypokalemia, and

Ecstasy
• "Ecstasy" is a common term for the ring-substituted form of metham-phetamine, also known as a "drug club" by teens and young adults.
• Ecstasy causes ADH secretion and water accumulation in the stomach and intestine by decreasing gastrointestinal (GI) motility. Hypo-natremia occurs due to excess water consumption and poor reabsorp-tion of the GI tract in the presence of elevated levels of ADH.
• Rapid correction of [Na+] is indicated in ecstasy-induced hypo-natremia.

Selective Serotonin Re-uptake Inhibitors
Selective serotonin re-uptake inhibitors (SSRIs) are by far the most of-ten-used medications for depression. Drugs such as sertraline, paroxe-tine, and duloxetine inhibit the re-uptake of serotonin and improve de-pression. Hyponatremia is due to drug-induced SIADH. Mechanisms include:
    (1) Stimulation of ADH secretion,
    (2) Extension of ADH action in the renal medulla,
    (3) Reset of the osmostat that lowers the ADH secretion threshold,
    (4) Interaction of SSRIs with other drugs through p450 enzymes, resulting in enhanced activity of ADH.

Exercise-Induced Hyponatremia
Exercise-induced hyponatremia (EIH) is a dangerous condition for marathon runners. Despite hyponatremia, the levels of ADH are raised. Factors that may precipitate hyponatremia.
    (1) Water consumption >3 L,
    (2) Body mass index <20 kg/m2,
    (3) Excess loss of sweat,
    (4) Nonsteroidal drugs,
    (5) Running time >4 h,
    (6) Postmarathon weight gain.
• Rapid correction of [Na+] is indicated in EIH.

Beer Potomania
• A condition marked by the history of substance dependence, hypo-natremia, signs and effects of water toxicity, protein malnutrition (chronic alcoholics), poor consumption of solutes, and little evidence of diuretic steroid usage.

- Generally, urine osmolality is lower than plasma osmolality but can approach 300 mOsm/kg H2O.
- At the initial presentation, ADH levels can be suppressed or high.
- The incidence of hyponatremia relies on the consumption of solute (e.g. protein, salt).
- Alcohols with or without hypokalemia are at significant risk for osmotic demyelination syndrome (ODS) with quick hyponatremia correction.
- Alcoholics with malnutrition and cirrhosis are also at higher risk for ODS.

Poor Oral Intake
- Poor oral intake of protein and salt, over days, usually occurs in elderly subjects with a slight decrease in glomerular filtration rate (GFR). This type of dietary pattern is called the "tea and toast" diet. It can induce hyponatremia with high water intake similar to that of beer or crash diet potomania with low solute intake.
- Protein and salt consumption enhance both hyponatremia and osmolality in the urine.
- Certain differences exist between subjects with beer potomania and "tea and toast" intake. Supply of adequate calories from beer, relatively severe hyponatremia
(98 mEq/L), hypokalemia, neurologic manifestations, and free water excretion with relatively normal GFR are common in beer potomania subjects compared to those on poor oral intake.

Postoperative Hyponatremia
- Common in hospitalized patients.
- Hypotonic fluids, drugs for pain and non-osmotic release of ADH are frequent causes.
- Hyponatremia can also occur with normal saline due to water accumulation in the presence of ADH. This is a concept called desalination. As normal saline is injected and intravascular volume is raised, the kidneys excrete NaCl with water accumulation, resulting in hyponatremia.
- Hysterectomy or prostate surgery can induce hyponatremia due to irrigation fluids like glycine.
- Young menstruating women are also at postoperative risk for ODS.

Hypokalemia and Hyponatremia

Hypokalemia is a rare cause of hyponatremia. The reason for hyponatremia is the movement of Na+ from ECF to the ICF compartment. At the same time, K+ goes out of the cell into the ECF compartment. This exchange maintains electroneutrality. Both hyponatremia and hypokalemia may occur occasionally. Repletion of K+ alone in the form of KCl may correct serum Na+ to the desired level without concomitant use of saline.

The following explains the Correction of serum [Na+].

- When KCl is administered, K+ and Cl− move into the cell, causing hyperosmolality. This draws water into the cell with a resultant rise in serum [Na+].
- Also, when K+ moves into the cell, H+ moves out of the cell. This H+ is buffered by bicarbonate and plasma protein, and the bicarbonate is converted into CO_2 and water. As a result, the plasma osmolality is decreased, and water moves into the cell. This raises serum [Na+].
- When saline is needed, the amount of Na+ required to achieve the desired level in a patient with both hyponatremia and hypokalemia should include both Na+ and K+ concentrations of the solution that should not exceed the total required amount.
- When severe hypokalemia (<2.5 mEq/L) is present with hyponatremia, only KCl may be needed to correct serum Na+ to the desired level.

Signs and Symptoms of Hyponatremia

Patients with plasma [Na+] >125 mEq/L are usually asymptomatic. Symptoms are mainly cognitive and are related to the intensity and rapidity of hyponatremia. Gastrointestinal signs such as nausea can be the first physiological manifestation accompanied by headache, yawning, lethargy, restlessness, dizziness, ataxia, and depressed deep tendon reflexes (Na+< 125 mEq/L). Patients with Accelerated hyponatremia develop seizures, coma, respiratory arrest, irreversible brain injury, and even death can occur.

Signs & Symptoms of Hyponatremia
Remember "**SALT LOSS**"
Seizures & Stupor
Abdominal cramping, attitude changes (confusion)
Lethargic
Tendon reflexes diminished, trouble concentrating (confused)
Loss of urine & appetite
Orthostatic hypotension, overactive bowel sounds
Shallow respirations (happens late due to skeletal muscle weakness)
Spasms of muscles

Approach to the Patient with Hyponatremia

Step 1. Calculate serum osmolality

Hypotonic hyponatremia is called true hyponatremia. Low serum osmolality rules out pseudo and hypertonic hyponatremia.

Step 2. Measure urine osmolality and na+ concentration

Urine osmolality differentiates low osmolality (<100 mOsm/kg H2O) from high osmolality (>100 mOsm/kg H2O) conditions.

Step 3. Estimate volume status

History

• Evaluate for fluid loss (diarrhea, vomiting).

• Review medicines, such as oral hypoglycemics, antihypertensives, antidepressants, etc.

• Review medical diseases, such as psychiatric illness, cancer, and cardiovascular disease.

• Check intravenous (IV) fluids for maintenance and medication use.

Physical Examination

• Vital signs with orthostatic changes.

• Examination of the neck, lungs, heart, and lower extremities for fluid status.

• Evaluation of mental status is extremely important.

Step 4: Classify Hypotonic Hyponatremia Into

1. Hypovolemic hyponatremia (comparatively more Na+ than water loss)

2. Hypervolemic hyponatremia (comparatively more water than Na+ gain)
3. Normovolemic hyponatremia (comparatively more water than Na+)

Step 5. Obtain pertinent laboratory tests
- Serum chemistry, uric acid, and lipid panel.
- Complete blood count.
- Fractional excretion of Na+, phosphate, and uric acid is often required.
- Check the liver, thyroid, and adrenal function tests.

Step 6. Know more about pseudo or factitious hyponatremia
- Occasionally [Na+] serum is low in patients with extreme hyperlipidemia or hyperproteinemia.
- Reduction in [Na+] is due to the displacement of serum water by excess lipid or protein, but the serum osmolality is normal.
- This condition is called pseudo hyponatremia.
- These people have no symptoms because their osmolality in the serum is normal.

Step 7. Hypertonic (translocational) hyponatremia
- Severe hyperglycemia also reduces serum [Na+] due to water transfers from intracellular to extracellular compartments (translocation).
- Serum [Na+] reduces by 1.6 mEq/L for each 100 mg/dL glucose above natural glucose level (i.e. 100 mg/dL). This corrective factor refers to glucose levels of up to 400 mg/dL. If the serum glucose content is >400 mg/dL, the serum [Na+] would decrease by 2.4 mEq/L.
- Due to hyperglycemia, serum osmolality is elevated, and the disorder is called hypertonic hyponatremia.
- Hyperglycemia correction also fixes hyponatremia.
- Mannitol, sucrose, glycerol, glycine, and maltose can also induce hypertonic hyponatremia.

Step 8. Rule out reasons other than glucose that increase plasma osmolality

Urea, ethanol, methanol, and ethylene glycol can also raise plasma osmolality. Calculation of the osmolar gap is useful. However, these solutes are inefficient osmolytes and are cell-permeable. They do not, however, induce the translocation of water.

Diagnosis of Hypotonic Hyponatremia

Urine osmolality is often >100 mOsm/kg H2O in all situations that cause hypotonic hyponatremia except for psychogenic polydipsia, beer potomania, and reset osmostat. Urinary Na is stated to be <10 mEq/L only in vomiting, diarrhea, and decompensated congestive heart failure (CHF), cirrhosis, and nephrotic syndrome. Acute kidney damage due to volume loss often causes low Na+ in the urinary tract. The fractional excretion of Na+ opposes the excretion of UNa.

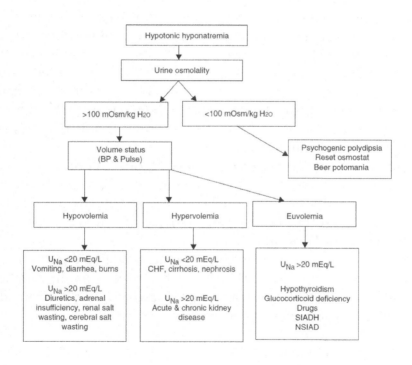

Brain Adaptation to Hyponatremia

Cell volume is maintained during extreme conditions of either hypo- or hypertonicity by adjusting its intracellular solute contents. If plasma osmolality is low, water flows into the brain, causing swelling of the brain and Edema. Astrocytes, rather than neurons, play a role in brain swelling. Blood flow to the brain decreases, leading to brain herniation. Since brain expansion is limited due to a solid skull, intracranial hypertension occurs, and neurological symptoms occur in a hyponatremic patient. However, symptoms fade progressively as the brain starts to respond to hyponatremia. The main adaptive process is the extrusion of $Na+$, $Cl-$, $K+$, and organic osmolytes (myositol, taurine, glycine, etc.) from the brain cells. This results in a decrease of intracellular osmolality, which inhibits further water passage into the cell. Subsequently, even in the case of extreme hyponatremia, the brain volume returns to baseline. This adaptation is nearly complete within 48 h. The clinician should keep this simple physiologic mechanism in mind while correcting hyponatremia. The slow correction will allow the extruded electrolytes and organic osmolytes to move back into the cell or synthesize the organic osmolytes to maintain normal cell volume. For this reason, the guidelines have suggested limits of correction (increase in $Na+$) for 24 and 48 h periods (see treatment). There are some factors that may impair brain adaptation to hyponatremia.

Complications of Untreated Chronic Hyponatremia

Mild chronic hyponatremia is not without its complications. Studies have shown cognitive dysfunction, falls, fractures, and osteoporosis in patients having serum $[Na+]$ between 126 and 134 mEq/L.

Management of Hyponatremia

Hyponatremia is classically categorized as acute (<48 h duration) or chronic (>48 h duration) and is further categorized as asymptomatic or symptomatic. In terms of treatment, this classification is essential. Therefore the treatment of hyponatremia
depends on four factors:

1. Severity of hyponatremia
2. Duration of hyponatremia
3. Signs and symptoms of hyponatremia
4. Volume status.

Treatment of Acute Symptomatic Hyponatremia

1. Acute symptomatic hyponatremia (seizures, respiratory failure, etc.) is a medical emergency.
2. Provide adequate oxygenation. Treat hypoxemia to prevent exacerbation of hyponatremic encephalopathy.
3. Patients at risk for acute symptomatic hyponatremia:
   a. Postoperative patients receiving hypotonic fluids
   b. Psychogenic polydipsic patients
   c. Patients taking ecstasy
   d. Marathon runners.
4. For the above patients, 3% NaCl is the fluid of choice because its infusion raises serum [Na+] to the desired level and prevents Cerebral Edema. Rarely, 5% of saline is required. Raise serum Na+ 6–8 mEq in 3–4 h. Rapid correction to higher than 8 mEq in 24 h may not be that harmful, particularly in patients with psychogenic polydipsia, patients taking ecstasy, and marathon runners. Water restriction should NEVER be used to treat symptomatic hyponatremia because it takes 24–72 h to increase Na+ by 5–6 mEq.
5. In all other symptomatic patients, 3% NaCl should also be used. Raise serum Na+ 1–2 mEq/h for 3 h equal to 6 mEq from baseline. Then hold 3% NaCl. If symptoms endure, give another bolus of 100 mL of 3% NaCl. The increase in serum Na+ is 6–8 mEq in a 24 h period in patients with no risk factors. In high-risk patients, the rate of correction should not exceed 6 mEq in a 24 h period.
6. The above correction rates can be achieved by giving 1–2 mL/kg/h or 100 mL boluses of 3% NaCl. Repeat these boluses two to three times as needed. Presuming no urine excretion of Na+, a bolus of 100 mL raises serum [Na+] by 1 mEq.
7. To prevent overcorrection, it is helpful to measure the amount of Na+ needed to reach the desired degree. If the patient weighs 70 kg and the serum [Na+] is 110 mEq/L, and you want to raise it to 116 mEq/L, use the following basic formula:

   Amount of Na+ needed = Total body water × desired Na$^+$ – actual Na$^+$

   1L of 3% NaCl comprises 513 mEq of Na+.

8. Remember that these measurements are based on the premise that the patient would not lose any Na+ in the urine. This cannot be achieved in conventional practice until the patient is anuric.

9. Therefore, measure urine volume and urine Na+ concurrently with serum Na+ every 2 h until the symptoms get better. Replace urinary loss of Na+ with either 3% or 0.9% saline, as required, to achieve the target Na+.

10. NEVER correct serum Na+ levels above 6–8 mEq in a 24 h period from baseline irrespective of the risk factor.

11. If symptoms persist after serum Na+ has risen by 6 mEq/L, look for another cause for the neurologic symptoms.

12. If the patient develops pulmonary congestion, administer furosemide 20–40 mg. With furosemide, the patient loses both electrolytes and water. However, the urine output generally exceeds input, resulting in a gradual increase in serum Na+ level.

13. If serum Na+ levels increase by > 10–12 mEq/L, administer DDAVP 1–2 µg IV with boluses of 5% dextrose in water (D5W) or 4–5 µg subcutaneously, and follow serum Na+ level. Repeat every 6–8 h until serum [Na+] decreases to the desired level (i.e., 6 mEq/L above baseline).

14. Do not raise serum [Na+] >18 mEq/L in a 48-h period.

Treatment of Chronic Symptomatic Hyponatremia

1. Note that overcorrection of serum [Na+] predisposes chronic hyponatremia patients to ODS.

2. In chronic hyponatremia patients, cerebral water content increases by only 10%.
Therefore, the correction should not exceed 10%.

3. Use 3% NaCl. Do not exceed 1 mEq/h.

4. The maximum rate of correction in a 24 h period should not exceed 6–8 mEq.

5. Once symptoms and signs improve, either water restriction or normal saline should be started with measurements of urine output, urine Na+ and K+ with replacement of these cations as needed.

6. In case of overcorrection, lowering of serum [Na+] by DDAVP and D5W is necessary to prevent ODS.

7. For fluid overload, furosemide can be given with 3% NaCl or normal saline.

8. Vaptan use also has been advocated before discharge.

A complication of Rapid Correction of Hyponatremia

- ODS, previously called central pontine myelinolysis, is a complication of treating both acute and chronic hyponatremia.
- It occurs due to a rapid increase in serum [Na+] of 8–12 mEq in patients with no risk factors or >6 mEq in patients with risk factors above baseline in a 24-h period.
- The possible mechanism is the slow recovery of brain osmolytes during the rapid correction of hyponatremia compared to the loss of these osmolytes during brain volume adaptation.
- As serum [Na+] is dramatically elevated, plasma osmolality becomes hypertonic to the brain, resulting in the transfer of water from the brain that contributes to myelinolysis.

Risk Factors

Several risk factors for the precipitation of ODS have been identified. These are:

1. Chronic hyponatremia
2. Serum [Na+] <105 mEq/L
3. Chronic alcoholism
4. Malnutrition
5. Hypokalemia
6. Severe liver disease
7. Elderly women on thiazide diuretics
8. Children
9. Menstruating women
10. Hypoxia
11. Seizures on presentation and overcorrection (>20 mEq/L in 24 h)

Treatment of Asymptomatic Chronic Hyponatremia

Asymptomatic chronic hyponatremia occurs due to Syndrome of Inappropriate Antidiuretic Hormone Secretion in Ambulatory Patients. In that case,

1. Treat the underlying cause of SIADH.

2. Restrict fluid, as mentioned earlier.

3. If the patient is noncompliant with fluid restriction, enhance Na+ and protein intake to increase solute and water excretion. Furosemide (40 mg) can be tried with high Na+ intake.

4. Pharmacologic therapy can be started in some patients. Demeclocycline at 300–600 mg twice daily induces nephrogenic diabetes insipidus. The drug takes 3–4 days to take affect. The major problem with demeclocycline is nephrotoxicity, and in particular cirrhotic patients develop acute kidney injury.

5. Osmotic diuresis (more water than Na+ excretion) can be induced in some patients with noncompliance to water restriction. Urea at doses 30–60 g can be effective. Polyuria, GI discomfort, and unpalatability are some of the adverse effects of Urea. Urea is usually mixed with orange juice to make it palatable.

6. Drugs such as lithium and V2 receptor antagonists (vaptans) can be used to suppress ADH action. Lithium (900–1,200 mg/day) can be used. However, it has a narrow therapeutic and toxic range. Polyuria and neurotoxicity are major adverse effects of lithium. Close monitoring of serum [Na+] is necessary as hypernatremia due to polyuria is rather common if fluid intake is not adequate.

7. Among vaptans, conivaptan (IV) and tolvaptan (oral) are available in the USA. Although clinical experience is limited, tolvaptan has been used with encouraging results. Vaptans cause water diuresis and, therefore, are called aquaretics. Na+ loss is negligible. It is safer to start the first dose in the hospital to follow the pattern of hyponatremia. Diuresis starts 2–4 h following 15 mg of tolvaptan intakeSerum [Na+] should be checked in 2–4 h, as Na+ response is

unpredictable. The dose can be increased to 30 or 60 mg at 24 h intervals. Allow free water intake, which may counteract an abrupt increase in serum [Na+]. Use tolvaptan only when serum [Na+] is <125 mEq/L. Avoid vaptans in patients with cirrhosis.

8. Conivaptan can be used to treat hyponatremia in neurosurgical patients with or without other therapies. Case reports and case series suggest that a single or multiple conivaptan doses (10–40 mg IV over a 30 min period or boluses) improved serum [Na+] by 4–6 mEq/L in 24 h. No significant adverse effects, including ODS, were observed. In one case report, the 22-year-old woman had a motor-vehicle accident and subsequently developed hyponatremia (128 mEq/L) due to SIADH. Due to suspicion of Cerebral Edema and decreased cerebral perfusion, the patient received a bolus of conivaptan (20 mg), and serum Na+ level increased from 128 to 148 mEq/L in 8 h and intracranial pressure dropped from 11–15 to 2 mmHg. Fortunately, no adverse events were noted with a rapid increase in serum Na+ levels. Thus, conivaptan can be used to treat hyponatremia in neurosurgical ICUs.

Treatment of General Causes of Hyponatremia
Pseudohyponatremia
- No specific treatment
- Treat underlying cause.
Hypertonic hyponatremia due to hyperglycemia
- Correct glucose with insulin. Normal saline for hypotension, followed by 0.45% saline to improve volume and hypernatremia
- In a hypotensive and hypernatremic patient, normal saline is hypotonic to plasma osmolality.
Diarrhea
- Normal saline. KCl, if hypokalemic
- Replace electrolyte loss in secretory diarrhea.
Vomiting
- Normal saline. KCl, if hypokalemia present
- Treat the cause.
Salt-losing syndromes
- Normal saline
- Follow other electrolytes.

Cerebral salt wasting
- Normal saline, fludrocortisone
- NaCl tablets in an outpatient setting.
CHF and cirrhosis
- Salt restriction, loop diuretics, water restriction for hyponatremia
- Vaptans (in CHF only), if water restriction fails and diuretic resistance develops
- Edema and hyponatremia improve. Monitor serum [Na+] frequently when tolvaptan is used.

Acute and chronic kidney injury
- Water restriction
- Follow serum creatinine.

Primary polydipsia
- Water restriction
- Treat underlying cause.

Hypothyroidism
- Thyroxine
- Follow thyroid function tests.

Glucocorticoid deficiency
- Hydrocortisone
- Follow serum [Na+] and blood pressure.

SSRIs
- Water restriction
- Do not use hydrochlorothiazide (HCTZ) concomitantly.

HCTZ
- Discontinue HCTZ. KCl alone is sufficient to raise serum [Na+] in mild hyponatremia. Use NaCl tablets
- Do not overcorrect the K+ deficit. Careful in using both normal saline and KCl.

Exercise-induced hyponatremia (symptomatic)
- 3% NaCl until serum [Na+] reaches 125 mEq/L or symptoms improve
- Avoid pure water intake >3 L and nonsteroidal drug use.

Low solute intake ("tea and toast" diet)
- Increase dietary salt and protein intake.
- Water restriction is helpful
- Follow urine osmolality
- Seen commonly in elderly subjects.

Beer potomania
- Dietary salt and protein
- Normal saline, as indicated
- Water restriction may help some patients
- Follow urine osmolality.

Postoperative hyponatremia (asymptomatic)
- Normal saline is treatment of choice
- Follow urine electrolytes and osmolality
- Avoid hypotonic solutions when serum [Na+] <138 mEq/L.
- Hold normal saline once euvolemia is achieved.

Hypernatremia

By definition, Hypernatremia is,
- Levels of serum or plasma [Na+] >145 mEq/L
- Hyperosmolality (serum osmolality >295 mOsm/kg H2O).

Hypernatremia can develop by a shortfall in total body water and/or a gain of Na+, or a combination of both.

Mechanisms of Hypernatremia

In a healthy individual, two mechanisms defend against hyper-natremia:
(1) thirst
(2) excretion of concentrated urine.

An increase in serum [Na+] and related to hyperosmolality creates thirst, and water intake lowers serum [Na+] to a normal level. By excreting concentrated urine, the kidneys try to conserve water. Thus, hypernatremia and hyperosmolality are prevented.

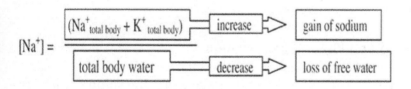

The Edelman equation shows the serum sodium concentration (Na$^+$) as a function of the total interchangeable sodium and potassium in the body, as well as the total body water.

Hypernatremia develops when patients:
- Cannot experience or respond to thirst
- Have no access to water
- Have salt loading
- Excretion of dilute urine with no or resistance to ADH.

Patients at Risk for Hypernatremia
- Elderly
- Children
- People with diabetes with uncontrolled glucose

- Patients with polyuria
- Hospitalized patients due to lack of ample free water intake or administration
- Osmotic diuretics (mannitol)
- Impaired water conservation due to concentrating inability
- Lactulose administration
- Normal or hypertonic saline administration
- Tube feedings or hyperalimentation
- Mechanical ventilation.

Approach to the Patient with Hypernatremia

Step 1: Estimate Volume Status

Based on volume status, classify hypernatremia into:
- Hypovolemic hypernatremia (comparatively more water than Na+ loss)
- Hypervolemic hypernatremia (comparatively more Na+ than water gain)
- Normovolemic or euvolemic Hypernatremia (water loss but with normal Na+ concentration).

Step 2: History and Physical Examination

History:
- Evaluate the quantity of water intake and urine volume. Identify the cause of water loss
- Infusions of hypertonic saline, hyperalimentation, or mannitol, including hyperglycemia for osmotic diuresis
- Obtain a history of diabetes, excessive sweating, or diarrhea
- Dietary history of high protein and electrolyte intake
- Medications such as lactulose, loop diuretics, lithium, and analgesics.

Physical Examination:
- Vital signs and orthostatic changes (very important and mandatory)
- Record body weight
- Examination of the neck, lungs, and heart for fluid overload and lower extremities for edema
- Evaluation of mental status is extremely important.

Step 3: Diagnosis of Hypernatremia

The most important tests, besides urine volume, are:
- Plasma and urine osmolality
- Urine Na+ and K+
- Other laboratory tests include serum K+, creatinine, BUN, and Ca2+ for assessment of renal function
- Brain imaging studies, if indicated.

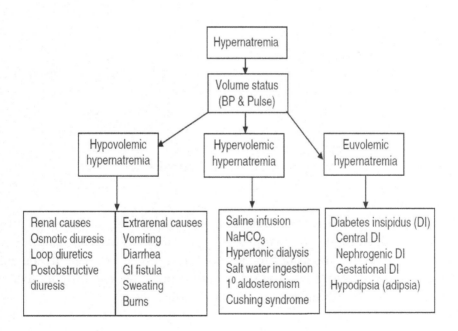

Volume status	Hypovo-lemic	Euvolemic	Hypervo-lemic
Orthostatic changes	yes	No	No
Urinary sodium U_{Na} (mEq/L)	>20 (renal) <20 (extrarenal)	>20	>20
Urine osmolality (mOsm/kg H_2O)	>100 (both renal and extrarenal)	<100 (central DI) >100 (nephrogenic DI)	>100
Edema	No	No	Yes

Brain Adaptation to Hypernatremia

When the level of serum [Na+] rises, the brain volume decreases due to the exit of water and electrolytes, causing a decrease in intracranial pressure. However, within a few hours, adaptive changes occur by moving water, electrolytes, and organic osmolytes into the brain, thereby returning brain volume to normal.

Signs and Symptoms of Hypernatremia

Mostly neurological due to the shrinkage of the brain and the tearing of brain vessels.

- Sudden Hypernatremia: nausea, vomiting, lethargy, irritability, and fatigue. These signs and symptoms can lead to seizures and coma.

- Chronic Hypernatremia (present for >1–2 days): fewer neurological signs and symptoms due to brain adaptation; however, fatigue, nystagmus, and impaired sensorium can be observed.

Hypernatremia (F.R.I.E.D. S.A.L.T.)
• Flushed skin (temperature)
• Restlessness (neuro excitability)
• Increased DTR's (neuro excitability)
• Edema
• Decreased urine output (dehydration)
• Sleepy (overworked system)
• Agitated (neuro excitability)
• Low-Grade Fever (diminished sweating)
• Thirsty (dehydration)

Other Consequences of Hypernatremia

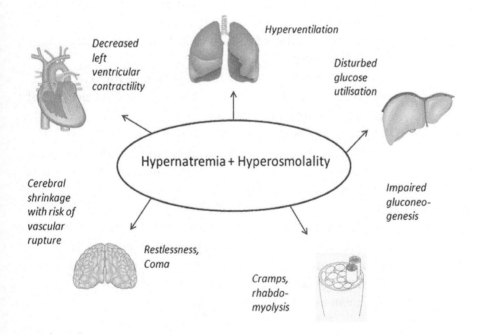

Decreased left ventricular contractility

Hyperventilation

Disturbed glucose utilisation

Cerebral shrinkage with risk of vascular rupture

Hypernatremia + Hyperosmolality

Impaired gluconeo-genesis

Restlessness, Coma

Cramps, rhabdo-myolysis

Specific Causes of Hypernatremia

Polyuria

Polyuric syndromes are the most important causes of hypernatremia. These syndromes cause diuresis of both water and solute (osmotic diuresis, Diabetes insipidus, both Central DI, nephrogenic DI, and gestational DI cause diuresis of the water; while hyperalimentation and infusion of hypertonic saline, glucose, and mannitol cause diuresis of the solute). At the same time, psychogenic polydipsia causes polyuria-related hyponatremia.

Central DI

- Central DI is due to the failure to synthesize or release ADH from the hypothalamus.
- Two types of central DI are: complete and partial.
- The thirst mechanism is intact in most, except in patients with craniopharyngiomas (postoperative).
- Urine osmolality is typically ≤100 mOsm/kg H2O of incomplete form.
- Distal nephron responds to the action of the ADH.
- Patients typically prefer ice or ice water, and nocturnal urinary complaints are usual.
- The cause is both congenital and acquired.
- Post-traumatic, postsurgical, metastatic tumors, granulomas, and CNS infections are the most common causes of acquired central DI.

Nephrogenic DI

- Nephrogenic DI is characterized as a tubular resistance to ADH despite an adequate plasma level of ADH.
- The thirst system is still intact.
- Urine osmolality is <300 mOsm/kg of H2O.
- Both causes are congenital and inherited.

There are two forms of congenital nephrogenic DI:

1. X-linked variant (90 percent of cases) due to loss of function mutation in the vasopressin 2 receptor. Males with this mutation are diagnosed with dehydration, hypernatremia, and hyperthermia as early as the first week of life. Mental and physical retardation and kidney dysfunction can occur as a result of a delayed diagnosis.
2. The second type either has an autosomal dominant or recessive inheritance (10 percent of cases). It is caused by the loss-of-function mutation of the AQP gene. Polyuria, dehydration, and hypernatremia are common. Carriers with the AQP gene mutation are at risk of thromboembolism due to elevated secretion of the von Willebrand factor, the carrier protein for factor VIII.

Treatment
- Treatment of both conditions requires hypotonic fluids to avoid dehydration.
- Hydrochlorothiazide, alone or in conjunction with amiloride or indomethacin, can help to reduce urine production.
- Phosphodiesterase inhibitors that prevent the degradation of cAMP and cGMP have been studied, with varying results.

Acquired Nephrogenic DI:
CKD, hypokalemia, protein malnutrition, hypercalcemia, sickle cell disease, lithium, or demeclocycline treatment are important causes of acquired nephrogenic diabetes insipidus.

Gestational DI
• Occurs during late pregnancy and settles after delivery.
• Caused by the degradation of vasopressin (ADH) by the enzyme vasopressinase, and the placenta produces this enzyme.
• Treatment is desmopressin (DDAVP), which is not reduced by vasopressinase.

Hypodipsic (Adipsic) Hypernatremia
Hypodipsic conditions are characterized by an absent or inadequate sensation of thirst, with decreased water intake despite water availability. It arises as a result of the complete or partial destruction of osmoreceptors for thirst.

Treatment of Hypernatremia

Treatment of Hypernatremia depends on six factors:

1. Correction of the underlying cause
2. Calculation of water deficit
3. Selection and route of fluid administration
4. Volume status
5. Onset of Hypernatremia (acute or chronic)
6. Rate of correction.

Correction of the Underlying Cause

Causes of Hypernatremia, such as diarrhea, hyperglycemia, diuretic use, hypokalemia, hypercalcemia, and saline or mannitol infusion, should be addressed and treated, if possible.

Calculation of Water Deficit

Administration of 3–4 mL/kg of electrolyte-free water can lower serum [Na+] by one mEq/L. Total water deficit can be calculated as weight in kilogram × milliliters to be administered (3 or 4 mL) × the difference between the actual and desired [Na+].

Selection and Route of Fluid Administration

Selection of fluid is based on blood pressure. If the patient is hypotensive, normal saline is the fluid of choice despite hypernatremia. Note that normal saline is relatively hypotonic in a patient with severe hypernatremia. If possible, oral intake of water is preferred to correct hypernatremia; however, most patients require IV administration. Fluids that are commonly used are D5W, 0.45%, or 0.225% saline. Infrequently, hemodialysis is used in patients with salt loading.

Volume Status

As mentioned previously, the estimation of volume status is extremely important to select the appropriate fluid.

Treatment of Acute Hypernatremia

• Prevention of Hypernatremia in hospitalized patients is important, as its development is mostly iatrogenic, resulting from the inadequate and inappropriate prescription of fluids to patients whose water deficits are large, and their thirst mechanism is impaired.

• Hypernatremia developed over hours due to salt-overload, or following hypothalamic-pituitary surgery, can be fully corrected with appropriate fluid (oral fluids or IV D5W or 0.225% saline) to the baseline value without causing cerebral edema because accumulated electrolytes (Na+, K+, and Cl–) are extruded from brain cells.
• The consequences of acute hypernatremia are shrinkage of brain cells and intracranial hemorrhage.
• The rate/pace of correction is 1 mEq/h.
• Administration of the volume includes the amount of water deficit and ongoing fluid losses (insensible loss and loss from other sources).

Treatment of Chronic Hypernatremia

• Hypernatremia developed 24–48 h later is considered chronic, and brain adaptation is complete. Therefore, slow correction is warranted.
• The rate/pace of correction is 6–8 mEq/L in a 24-h time with full correction in 2–3 days.
• Studies in children showed that outcomes were better when the rate of correction was ≤0.5 mEq/h.

Treatment of Specific Causes

Hypovolemic Hypernatremia
• Administer normal saline until hemodynamic stability is established.
• Once the patient is euvolemic, give D5W or 0.45% saline to correct the water deficit and ongoing water losses.

Hypervolemic Hypernatremia
• Not uncommon in intensive care units because of saline or mannitol infusion.
• Administer loop rather than thiazide diuretics.
• Use of loop diuretics may increase water deficit; therefore, the need for free water is increased.
• In some situations, consider hemodialysis.

Normovolemic (Euvolemic) Hypernatremia (Central DI)
• DDAVP is the drug of choice for central DI.
• Available as a nasal spray or oral form.
• Use the lowest dose of 5–10 μg nasally or 0.1 or 0.2 mg orally at bedtime to avoid nocturia and hyponatremia.

• Duration of therapy varies according to the cause of central DI. The idiopathic disease requires permanent use, and the acquired form may require therapy transiently.

• Other drugs such as chlorpropamide, carbamazepine, or clofibrate can be used in patients with partial central DI, as they can stimulate ADH release.

• Induction of mild volume depletion with salt restriction and thiazide use (25 mg daily) can be effective in some patients with central DI, but more effective in nephrogenic DI.

• Congenital DI patients should receive enough water to prevent dehydration.

• Thiazide diuretics may be helpful.

• Removal of the cause, water intake, thiazide, and amiloride are the mainstay of therapy in acquired nephrogenic DI.

Hypernatremia in the Elderly

Chronic hypotonic hypernatremia is very frequent in patients of long-term care facilities. Reasons that account for hypernatremia in the elderly:

(1) reduced water consumption due to inaccessibility of water.

(2) lack of appetite or relative hypodipsia.

(3) consumption of loop diuretics.

(4) additional protein-intake and urea-induced water loss.

Hypertonic hypernatremia is not very common unless the patient requires a repeated infusion of saline or $NaHCO_3$.

Euvolemic Hypernatremia is also common due to drugs such as lithium. Elderly participants have decreased ability to concentrate urine, relative to young people.

Impaired mental state (lethargy, confusion) is typical with moderate hypernatremia, and seizures and coma can occur with extreme hypernatremia.

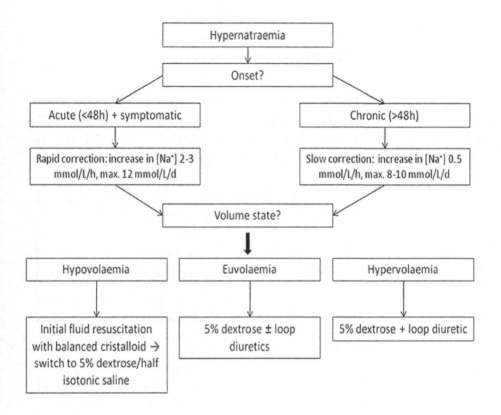

Important to remember
- Drugs that can increase serum sodium levels include anabolic steroids, angiotensin, bicarbonate, carbenoxolone, cisplatin, corticotropin, cortisone, gamma globulin, and mannitol.
- Substances that may reduce serum sodium levels include amphotericin B, bicarbonate, cathartics (excessive use), chlorpropamide, chlorthalidone, diuretics, ethacrynic acid, fluoxetine, furosemide, laxatives (excessive use), methyclothiazide, metolazone, nicardipine, quinethazone, theophylline (IV infusion), thiazides, and triamterene.
- Specimens should never be obtained above the IV line due to the potential for dilution when the specimen and the IV solution are mixed in the collection container, incorrectly reducing the outcome. The probability of contaminating the sample with the substance of interest contained in the IV solution is also falsely increasing.

Chapter 4
Serum potassium

Potassium (K+) is the primary intracellular cation in the body. Inside the cells [K+] is 140–150 mEq/L; it is 3.5–5 mEq/L in the blood. The serum contains a slightly higher concentration of K+ than plasma because K+ is released from red blood cells during clot formation.

Serum	SI Units (Conversion Factor X1)
Newborn	3.7–5.9 mmol/L or mEq/L
Infant	4.1–5.3 mmol/L or mEq/L
Child	3.4–4.7 mmol/L or mEq/L
Adult	3.5–5.0 mmol/L or mEq/L

Also, a high concentration of K+ within the cell is necessary to preserve the resting membrane potential for cellular excitability & contraction. The high intracellular concentration of K+ is sustained by the Na/K-ATPase found in all cell membranes of animal cells. A variety of hormones influences this enzyme's activity. Electrolyte concentrations and the equilibrium is regulated by the exchange of oxygen and carbon dioxide in the lungs, the absorption, secretion and excretion of many compounds by the kidneys, and the secretion of hormones by endocrine glands.

- K+ is important for the propagation of electrical impulses in the cardiac and skeletal muscles.
- It also acts in enzymatic reactions that transform glucose into energy as well as amino acids into proteins.
- Potassium helps to maintain the acid-base balance and has a significant and inverse relation to pH: a pH decrease of 0.1 increases the potassium level by 0.6 mEq / L.

The kidney is the main route for the excretion of K+. Generally, the excretion of K+ in the urine, or kaliuresis, matches the dietary intake. The other path for the excretion of K+ is the colon. K+ excretion by the colon is increased under conditions of reduced renal activity.

Renal Handling of K+ Transport

Renal handling of K+ involves filtration, reabsorption, and secretion. Most of the filtered K+ is reabsorbed in the proximal nephron, while the distal segments of the nephron secrete the K+ in the urine.

Proximal Tubule

The glomerulus freely filters K+. The proximal tubule absorbs about 60–80 percent of this purified K+. K+ reabsorption is largely passive and occurs through a K+ transporter coupled with Na+ and water transport. Volume expansion and osmotic diuretics (e.g. mannitol) impede the passive diffusion of Na+-coupled K+ transport.

Loop of Henle

Both K+ secretion and reabsorption occur in this portion of the nephron. K+ crosses the later section of the proximal tubule and the thin descending limb of the Henle loop. The thick ascending limb of the loop of Henle actively re-absorbs K+.

Distal Tubule

Approximately 10% of the diluted K+ enters the distal tubule. The K+ secretion occurs in this section due to low luminal Cl– and high luminal Na+ concentrations. In this section, the K/Cl co-transporter is responsible for the K+ secretion. K+ secretion also happens via the ROMK channel.

Connecting Tubule

The connecting tubule cells' apical membrane contains Na+ (ENaC) and K+ (ROMK) conductance channels. The entry of Na+ via the ENaC creates a lumen-negative potential difference, promoting K+ secretion via ROMK. The connecting tubule cells secrete K+ faster than the rate at which it is excreted in the urine. K+ secretion is sensitive to aldosterone

Cortical Collecting Duct

The collecting duct is known to be the major K+ secretion site. There are two groups of cells in this segment: the primary cells and the intercalated cells. Primary cells are the key cells for K+ secretion. The intercalated A-type cell is involved in K+ reabsorption. K+ reabsorbs this cell in exchange for H+ secretion via H/K-ATPase. One HCO3– is produced for each H+ secreted. The H/K-ATPase can also participate in the acid-base balance.

Hypokalemia

Hypokalemia is characterized as a serum of [K+] <3.5 mEq/L.

The major causes of hypokalemia can be divided into five primary categories:

(1) dietary intake

(2) K+ cell uptake (transcellular)

(3) loss through the renal system

(4) loss through the gastrointestinal tract

(5) skin loss.

Causes of Hypokalemia and the Mechanism

1. Dietary:

- Low-K+ diet. Combination of low dietary K+ and its obligatory loss in urine
- Eating disorders. Low oral intake and total body K+ depletion
- High-carbohydrate intake with alcohol. Low K+ intake and shift into cells.

2. Transcellular distribution:

- Insulin Shift of K+ into cells
- β2-Agonists (albuterol, clenbuterol)
- Alkalosis
- Theophylline, caffeine
- B12 injections cause consumption of K+ in protein synthesis
- Familial hypokalemic periodic paralysis. Mutation in the gene encoding the α1-subunit of skeletal muscle L-type Ca2+ channel (60–70% of cases), or mutation in the gene encoding the skeletal muscle Na+ channel
- Thyrotoxic hypokalemic periodic paralysis. Hyperthyroidism.

3. Renal loss:

- Drugs (diuretics other than K+-sparing diuretics, penicillins, amphotericin B, lithium, cisplatin, licorice, gentamicin, amikacin, tobramycin, mineralocorticoids, cetuximab)
- Renal K+ wasting
- Hypokalemic-hypertensive disorders
- Activation of the renin–AII–aldosterone
- Malignant hypertension
- Renovascular hypertension

- Renin-secreting tumors. Excess aldosterone production by adrenals
- Primary aldosteronism. Mutation in ENaC
- Liddle syndrome. Excess aldosterone production
- Glucocorticoid-remediable aldosteronism. Deficiency of 11β-hydroxysteroid dehydrogenase enzyme
- Apparent mineralocorticoid excess syndrome. Mutation in the mineralocorticoid receptor
- Activating mutations of the mineralocorticoid receptor
- Deficiency of 11β- and 17α-hydroxylase enzymes
- Congenital adrenal hyperplasia Renal K+ wasting
- Hypokalemic-normotensive disorders
- Renal tubular acidosis (types 1 and 2) Renal K+ wasting
- Bartter syndrome. Mutations in Na/K/2Cl co-transporter and ROMK channel
- Gitelman syndrome. Mutation in distal tubule Na/Cl co-transporter
- Hypomagnesemia Renal K+ wasting
- Cushing's syndrome. Same as above.

4. Gastrointestinal loss
- Diarrhea K+ loss in stools
- Vomiting Renal K+ wasting.

5. Skin loss
- Excessive heat. Skin loss
- Strenuous exercise. Renal loss.

Hypokalemia causes
"Many Diuretics Generate Reversible Hypokalemia"
• **M**ineralocorticoids, e.g. fludrocortisone, exogenous
• **D**iuretics
• **G**astrointestinal loss – vomiting, diarrhea
• **R**edistribution – insulin, beta2 agonists, alkalosis
• **H**yper-aldosteronism

Diagnosis

Step 1
- History and physical examination are essential.
- BP is extremely important, as high or low BP gives clues to the etiology of hypokalemia.

Step 2
- Rule out pseudohypokalemia.
- Patients with leukemia and leukocyte count > 100,000/ μl can present with hypokalemia because of K+ uptake by these leukocytes.

Step 3
- Exclude poor oral intake and transcellular distribution of K+.
- Note that the total body K+ is normal in conditions of transcellular distribution.

Step 4
- In true hypokalemia, total body K+ is depleted.
- Determination of 24 h urine Na+ and K+ concentration is important.
- Spot urine K+ determination is not useful, as K+ excretion is variable in the day. If 24 h urine collection is not feasible, the urine K+/creatinine ratio in spot urine can be performed. A urine ratio <15 mEq/g creatinine suggests extrarenal loss, whereas a ratio >200 mEq/g creatinine suggests renal loss.
- Normal urine K+ in HypoPP and others that cause transcellular distribution.
- If urinary Na+ is < 100 mEq/day and urinary K+ <20 mEq/day (i.e., 24 h urine), suspect extrarenal losses from either the gastrointestinal tract or the skin.
- Note that K+ loss from diarrhea, malabsorption, or fistulas, causes normal anion-gap metabolic acidosis, instead of hypokalemic metabolic alkalosis due to vomiting.

Step 5
- If urinary Na+ is > 100 mEq/day and urinary K+ >20 mEq/day (i.e., 24 h urine), suspect renal loss.
- At this time, the determination of BP most likely establishes the diagnosis of hypokalemia.

- High BP and high plasma renin and aldosterone levels suggest malignant HTN, renovascular HTN, or renin-secreting tumors.
- High plasma aldosterone and low renin levels are characteristic of primary aldosteronism.
- Determine serum HCO3– in patients with hypokalemia and normal BP.
- Low serum HCO3 – suggests renal tubular acidosis.
- High serum HCO3– suggests metabolic alkalosis.
- In patients with metabolic alkalosis, the determination of urinary Cl– distinguishes renal from extrarenal causes of hypokalemia. Urine Cl– <10 mEq/L is suggestive of extrarenal loss, whereas > 10 mEq/L indicates a renal loss.

Tests to Confirm Hypokalemia
- Serum potassium measurement
- ECG
- If not evident clinically, 24-hour urinary potassium excretion and serum magnesium concentration.

Blood testing:
Hypokalemia can be observed during routine serum electrolyte tests. It should be suspected in individuals with typical ECG changes or muscular manifestations and risk factors verified by blood tests.

ECG
Cardiac effects of hypokalemia are usually minimal until serum potassium concentrations are < 3 mEq/L (< 3 mmol/L). Hypokalemia causes:
- Sagging of the ST segment,
- Depression of the T wave,
- Elevation of the U wave.

With evident hypokalemia, the T wave is increasingly smaller, and the U wave is becoming higher. Often a flat or positive T wave merges with a positive U wave, mistaken for QT prolongation.

Hypokalemia can cause premature ventricular beats and premature atrial contractions, ventricular and supraventricular tachyarrhythmias, and second or third-degree atrioventricular blocks. Such arrhythmias become more extreme with extremely serious hypokalemia; finally, ventricular fibrillation can occur. Patients with severe pre-existing heart failure, and digoxin users, are at risk of cardiac conduction disorders related to even moderate hypokalemia.

Diagnosis of Cause

1. The cause of hypokalemia is generally obvious from the history (in particular the history of the medications used); the clinical index of suspicion for the disorder is high:

- Drug screen in urine and/or serum for diuretics, amphetamines, and other sympathomimetic stimulants
- Serum renin, aldosterone, and cortisol
- 24-hour urine aldosterone, cortisol, sodium, and potassium
- Pituitary imaging to evaluate for Cushing syndrome
- Adrenal imaging to evaluate for adenoma
- Evaluation for renal artery stenosis
- Enzyme assays for 17-beta hydroxylase deficiency
- Thyroid function studies in patients with tachycardia
- Serum anion gap (e.g. to detect toluene toxicity).

2. After ruling out acidosis and other intracellular potassium shift causes, 24-hour urinary potassium and serum magnesium concentrations should be assessed.
3. Extrarenal (GI) potassium deficiency or reduced potassium intake is suspected in persistent inexplicable hypokalemia when renal potassium excretion is < 15 mEq/L (< 15 mmol/L).
4. Excretion of Na+ > 15 mEq/L (< 15 mmol/L). Indicates a renal source of potassium loss.
5. Unexplained hypokalemia with elevated renal potassium output and hypertension indicates an aldosterone secreting tumor or Liddle syndrome.

6. Unspecified hypokalemia with elevated renal potassium loss and normal blood pressure indicate Bartter Syndrome or Gitelman Syndrome, but hypomagnesemia, surreptitious vomiting, and diuretic misuse are more frequent, and should therefore be considered.

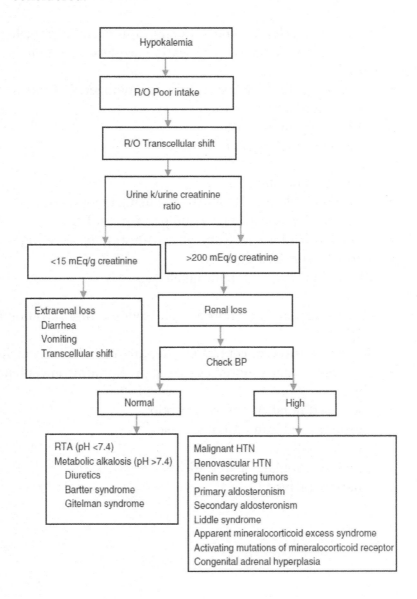

Clinical Manifestations

The clinical manifestations of hypokalemia are mostly neuromuscular and cardiac, which warrant immediate attention. Also, hypokalemia causes several metabolic and renal effects.

Clinical and physiologic manifestations of hypokalemia:

Neuromuscular
- Skeletal muscle: weakness, tetany, cramps, paralysis (flaccid)
- Smooth muscle: ileus, constipation, urinary retention.

Cardiovascular
- Abnormal EKG changes (U waves, prolonged Q-T interval, ST depression) and arrhythmias
- Abnormal contractility
- Potentiation of digitalis toxicity.

Metabolic
- Decreased insulin release
- Abnormal tolerance to glucose, causing diabetes
- Impaired hepatic glycogen and protein synthesis
- Decreased aldosterone and growth-hormone secretion
- Growth retardation
- Maintenance of metabolic alkalosis.

Renal
- Reduced renal blood flow as well as glomerular filtration rate (GFR)
- Impaired urine concentration (nephrogenic diabetes insipidus)
- Increased renal ammonia genesis, precipitating encephalopathy
- Increased renal HCO_3 reabsorption
- Chronic tubulointerstitial disease
- Cyst formation
- Proximal tubular vacuolization
- Rhabdomyolysis.

Hypokalemia (7 L's)
• Leg Cramps (decreased movement of K+)
• Lethal Cardiac Changes*
• Low and Slow Digestion (poor nerve conduction)
• Lethargic (poor nerve conduction)
• Low Amplitude DTR's (poor nerve conduction)
• Limp Muscles (poor nerve conduction)
• Low Shallow Respirations (poor nerve conduction)

Treatment

Treatment of hypokalemia depends on the following factors:

Severity

Mild to moderate hypokalemia (3–3.5 mEq/L) can be treated with oral KCl (40– 80 mEq/day). The oral route is the ideal way of administering KCl. Severe hypokalemia (< 2.5 mEq/L) can be life-threatening in a patient with cardiac disease and warrants immediate treatment. Intravenous (IV) administration of KCl is preferred to oral administration. Generally, 10–20 mEq of KCl in 100 mL of normal or one-half normal saline given over an hour is considered safe via the peripheral vein. Higher concentrations of KCl may lead to hyperkalemia, pain, and sclerosis of peripheral veins. KCl should not be given with dextrose solution for initial therapy because of the exacerbation of dextrose-induced hypokalemia through insulin release.

Underlying Cause

- If hypokalemia is due to the cellular shift, treating underlying causes is preferred.
- However, if severe weakness, paresis, or paralysis occurs, IV administration of KCl (10 mEq/h) should be given with EKG and plasma K+ monitoring.
- If the cellular shift is caused by thyrotoxicosis or excessive β-adrenergic, a nonselective β-blocker, such as propranolol, should be given. Causes of diarrhea should be sought and treated appropriately.

- Long-term use of K+-sparing diuretics is recommended for certain diseases.

Degree of K+ Depletion

It is not easy to estimate total body K+ depletion because it is largely stored in the muscle. As muscle mass decreases with age in both males and females, more in the former, everybody does not have the same weight. Total body K+ depletion should be individualized.

Treatment includes oral KCl alone or a combination of KCl and K+-sparing diuretics. Frequent monitoring of serum [K+] is indicated to avoid hyperkalemia.

Important to remember:
o Check for Magnesium
o Check potassium in Urine -- Is the Kidney doing its work?
o If not, BP is high or not? Hyper-aldosteronism or not? Primary vs. Secondary Hyperaldosteronism
o Do EKG
o Plasma K is more precise than serum K
o KCl: Only given via central line
o K-Gluconate: Can be given through peripheral access.

Hyperkalemia

Hyperkalemia is characterized as a serum level of [K+] >5.5 mEq/L. Hyperkalemia can be lethal if it is not recognized and treated promptly.

True hyperkalemia is caused by an

- excessive exogenous load of K+
- a decrease in cellular uptake
- a massive release following cell lysis
- a decrease in renal excretion
- Several drugs also cause hyperkalemia.

Pseudohyperkalemia refers to a phenomenon in which K+ is released from cells during venipuncture after sustained use of a tourniquet in the arm. Hemolysis of red blood cells and elevated numbers of white blood cells (>100,000 cells) and platelets (>1,000,000 platelets) also release K+ and induce pseudohyperkalemia. A benign type of familial pseudohyperkalemia also occurs due to the displacement of K+ from the blood cell. This condition has been identified in some families.

Causes of Hyperkalemia

1. *Exogenous intake*

- Oral. Excess oral intake High K+—containing foods (fruits, salt substitutes, KCl supplements, riverbed clay, burnt match heads, raw coconut juice)
- Herbal medications (horsetail, noni juice, dandelion, alfalfa)
- Endogenous K+ release from cell lysis
- Gastrointestinal bleeding
- Hemolysis
- Exercise
- Catabolic states
- Red cell transfusion
- Rhabdomyolysis
- Tumor lysis syndrome
- Thalidomide.

2. Transcellular shift (transfer of K+ from ICF to ECF)

- Insulin deficiency. Decreased cell uptake
- Hyperglycemia and hyperosmolality. Movement of K+ from ICF to ECF compartment by solvent drag β-Adrenergic blockers (propranolol, labetalol, carvedilol)
- Inhibit cellular K+ uptake and also inhibition of the renin–AII–aldosterone axis
- Digoxin causes Inhibition of Na/K-ATPase
- Chinese medicines (Dan Shen, Asian ginseng, Chan Su, Lu-Shen-Wan) cause inhibition of Na/K-ATPase
- Herbal remedies prepared from foxglove (Digitalis), lily of the valley, yewberry (Taxus), oleander, red squill, dogbane, toad skin also cause inhibition of Na/K-ATPase
- Succinylcholine K+ efflux from skeletal muscle via K+ channels
- Arginine, lysine, ε-aminocaproic acid K+ efflux from ICF to ECF
- Acute metabolic mineral acidosis (HCl or citric acid) causes K+ efflux from ICF to ECF
- Hyperkalemic periodic paralysis. Mutations in skeletal muscle Na+-channel.

3. Decreased renal excretion

- Advanced renal failure (CKD 5) and decreased delivery of filtrate to the distal tubule
- Diminished ability to secrete K+
- Hypoaldosteronism
- Addison's disease. Lack of glucocorticoid production
- Congenital adrenal hyperplasia 21α-hydroxylase deficiency
- Pseudohypoaldosteronism type I (PHA I). Autosomal dominant form: mutations in the mineralocorticoid receptor
- Autosomal recessive form: mutations in all subunits of ENaC
- Pseudohypoaldosteronism type II (PHA II). Mutations in "with no lysine" (WNK) 1 and 4 kinases
- Syndrome of hyporeninemic hypoaldosteronism

- Many diseases (diabetes, lupus, multiple myeloma, tubulointerstitial disease, AIDS) are associated with hyporeninemic hypoaldosteronism.

4. *Drugs*

- ACE inhibitors, ARBs, renin inhibitors, NSAIDs, COX-2 inhibitors, heparin, ketoconazole; all of these decrease aldosterone synthesis
- Amiloride, triamterene, trimethoprim, pentamidine. Block ENaC
- Spironolactone, eplerenone. Block aldosterone receptors
- Drospirenone. A progestin derived from spironolactone (used as a combined oral contraceptive)
- Cyclosporine, tacrolimus. (1) Hyporeninemic hypoaldosteronism, (2) block K+ channels in the distal nephron, (3) inhibit Na/K-ATPase, (4) inhibit ROMK channel, (5) increase Cl− shunt in DCT
- Cocaine, statins. Indirect effect by causing rhabdomyolysis.

Diagnosis
Step 1

• Check electrocardiogram (EKG), as hyperkalemia is an emergency. If there are no EKG abnormalities, proceed to step 2.
EKG changes in hyperkalemia. A normal EKG is also shown for comparison. The earliest change in hyperkalemia is the peaked (tented) T wave. With an increase in plasma [K+], the QRS complex widens, the P wave disappears, and finally, a sine wave pattern appears, leading to asystole.

Step 2

History:

• Inquire about diet and dietary supplements.

• Check medications that cause hyperkalemia.

• Review risk factors and disease conditions that predispose to hyper-kalemia.

Factors and conditions that predispose to hyperkalemia:

- CKD
- AKI
- Congestive heart failure and other conditions with decreased effective arterial blood volume
- Diabetes
- Volume depletion
- Elderly subjects
- White race
- Metabolic acidosis
- Dietary intake of foods and medications that contain K+
- Concomitant use of ACE-Is, ARBs, or renin inhibitors with the following drugs:
1. K+-sparing drugs
2. NSAIDs
3. β-Adrenergic blockers
4. Cyclosporine or tacrolimus
5. Heparin
6. Ketoconazole
7. Trimethoprim
8. Amiloride
9. Pentamidine.

Physical Examination

• Check blood pressure, pulse rate, and orthostatic blood pressure changes if indicated.

• Evaluate respiratory status for any weakness.

• Evaluate volume status.

• Evaluate muscle tenderness (rhabdomyolysis) and muscle weakness.

Step 3

• Obtain serum chemistry, complete blood count, and ABG (if needed).

• Measure UK/U-Creatinine ratio. The expected ratio in a patient with hyperkalemia and normal renal function is >200 mEq/g or >20 mmol/mmol. This ratio will be low in patients with decreased K+ excretion (CKD, volume-depleted, or hyporeninemic hypoaldosteronism patients). A 24-h urine collection for K+ excretion is needed for such patients.

• Establish true hyperkalemia after excluding pseudohyperkalemia and transcellular shift of K+. A UK/UCreatinine ratio far less than 200 mEq/g is suggestive of transcellular distribution.

• Obtain estimated GFR. Based on the estimated GFR, rule out defective K+ excretion.

• Obtain plasma aldosterone and renin levels. Obtain plasma cortisol levels as indicated.

• Delineate the cause of hyperkalemia.

Clinical Manifestations

Like hypokalemia, hyperkalemia also causes neuromuscular, cardiac, and metabolic effects.

Neuromuscular

- Muscle weakness due to reduced membrane potential caused by a reduction in the ratio of intracellular to extracellular [K+]
- Paralysis (ascending). Reduction in membrane potential from −90 mV to threshold potential, causing generation of an action potential.

Cardiac (EKG changes related to serum [K+])

- Serum K+ level 5.5–6.5 mEq/L = Peaked T waves with a narrow base
- Serum K+ level 6.5–8.0 mEq/L = Peaked T waves, prolonged PR interval, widening of QRS complex

- Serum K+ level > 8.0 mEq/L = Absence of P waves, further widening of QRS complex, bundle branch blocks, sine wave, ventricular fibrillation, asystole.

Metabolic

- Hyperchloremic (non-anion gap)
- Metabolic acidosis with hyperkalemia (hyperkalemic distal renal tubular acidosis)
- Urinary tract obstruction is the major cause. Decreased H+ secretion due to decreased cortical and medullary collecting duct H-ATPase activity. Urine pH is alkaline. However, combined hyperkalemic distal renal tubular acidosis, with low aldosterone, has been reported
- Type 4 renal tubular acidosis (RTA)
- Occurs in diseases and conditions with hyporeninism and hypoaldosteronism. Urine pH is usually acidic. The major defect is the suppression of NH4+ synthesis by hyperkalemia
- Drugs that cause aldosterone resistance also induce type 4 RTA.

Hyperkalemia (M.U.R.D.E.R.)
- **M**uscle weaknesses (poor nerve conduction)
- **U**rine production low or absent (dehydration)
- **R**espiratory failure (muscle weakness)
- **D**ecreased cardiac contractility (slows sodium and calcium entrance into the cell)
- **E**arly signs of twitching, and late signs of flaccidity (poor nerve conduction)
- **R**hythm changes

Treatment

Acute Treatment

Hyperkalemia is an acute emergency. Its management depends on serum [K+] and EKG changes. In many cases, hyperkalemia without EKG changes warrants treatment. The goals of acute therapy are threefold: (1) counteracting the membrane effects of hyperkalemia;

(2) promoting cellular uptake of K+; (3) removing K+ from the body slowly by cation exchange resin (sodium polystyrene sulfonate, Kayexalate) or a new approved nonabsorbable polymer (patiromer) or rapidly by hemodialysis using either a 1 or 2 mEq/L K+ dialysate bath. Kayexalate should be used cautiously, as when used on its own or in sorbitol, it can cause bowel necrosis. It should not be used in individuals with GI problems such as constipation, ischemic colitis, intestinal vascular atherosclerosis, and inflammatory bowel disease. Recently, two new oral K+-binding drugs have been introduced:

- patiromer (Veltassa, Relypsa)
- sodium zirconium cyclosilicate (ZS-9).

Patiromer is a nonabsorbable polymer that binds K+ in exchange for Ca2+. It binds K+ throughout the GI tract but preferentially in the distal colon. Patiromer reduces serum K+ levels in patients with CKD, cardiovascular disease, and diabetes on ACE-Is or ARBs and is well tolerated. GI-related adverse effects are most common with patiromer. ZS-9 is under the FDA review process and is effective in lowering serum K+ levels. It binds to K+ in exchange for Na+ and H+ ions. It is 125% more selective for K+ than kayexalate.

The list of different drugs/agents is as following:

Antagonism of membrane effects

Calcium gluconate (10%)

- dose: 10–20 mL
- onset of effect: 1–3 min
- duration of action: 30–60 min
- mechanism: Counteracts the membrane effects of K+.

Hypertonic (3%) saline

- dose: 50 mL
- onset of effect: Immediate
- duration of action: Unknown

- mechanism of action: Membrane antagonism.

Promote cellular uptake

Insulin and glucose

- dose: 20–50 g of glucose +10–20 U of rapid-acting insulin
- onset of effect: <30 min
- duration of action: 4–6 h
- mechanism of action: K+ uptake by cells.

$NaHCO_3$ (only when significant acidosis is present)

- dose: 44–88 mEq
- onset of effect: 5–10 min
- duration of action: 1–6 h
- mechanism of action: K+ uptake by cells.

Albuterol

- dose: 10–20 mg by nebulizer
- onset of effect: 15–20 min
- duration of action: 2–3 h
- mechanism of action: K+ uptake by cells.

Salbutamol

- dose: 10 mg by nebulizer
- onset of effect: 15–20 min
- duration of action: 2 h
- mechanism of action: K+ uptake by cells

Removal of K+ from body

Kayexalate (sodium polystyrene sulfonate) in 30% sorbitol (cation exchange resin)

- dose: Oral (30–45 g) or enema (50–100 g)
- onset of effect: ≥ 2 h
- duration of action: 2–6 h
- mechanism of action: Exchange of Na+ for K+.

Patiromer

- dose: Oral (8.4 g in water) once or twice
- onset of effect: >4 h
- duration of action: 24 h
- mechanism of action: Exchange of Ca2+ for K+.

Hemodialysis

- onset of effect: Immediate
- duration of action: 2–8 h
- mechanism of action: Immediate removal of K+ from ECF.

Chronic Treatment

• Patients with diabetes, tubulointerstitial disease, heart failure, and CKD of stage 4–5 are at risk for hyperkalemia.

• Estimate GFR and inquire about diet and dietary supplements.

• Review all the medications, including over-the-counter medications.

• Patients with chronic hyperkalemia have a defect (low lumen-negative voltage in the distal nephron) in eliminating their daily intake of K+ until they develop a new steady state.

• After a steady-state, they excrete their intake of K+ very slowly at the expense of higher plasma [K+].

• Use a loop diuretic (furosemide) or a thiazide diuretic, depending on GFR, to increase the delivery of Na+ to the distal nephron to increase the excretion of K+.

• Use kayexalate judiciously, if necessary.

• Alternatively, patiromer 8.4 g mixed in water can be taken once daily with food and 3 h before or 3 h after ingestion of all other medications.

• Use loop diuretics and/or fludrocortisone (0.05–0.1 mg orally) for patients with hyporeninemic hypoaldosteronism. Taper fludrocortisone as needed.

• Use NaHCO3 tablets to correct acidosis.

• In a patient with heart failure, use low doses of an ACE-I or ARB (do not use both). Follow serum creatinine and [K+] in 3–5 days. If creatinine increases by >30% and K+ are 6.0 mEq/L, hold ACE-I or ARB. If both measurements remain stable, repeat them in 7–14 days. If spironolactone is required, start with 12.5 mg, and go up to 25 mg/day. Some authors prefer to go up to 100 mg/day.

Chapter 5
Serum Calcium

General Features
Calcium (Ca2+) is the most abundant divalent ion in the body. Approximately 1.2 – 1.3 kg of Ca2+ is present in a 70 kg individual, mainly stored in bones.

Age	Conventional Units	SI Units (Conversion Factor X0.25)
Cord	8.2–11.2 mg/dL	2.05–2.80 mmol/L
0–10 d	7.6–10.4 mg/dL	1.90–2.60 mmol/L
11 d–2 y	9.0–11.0 mg/dL	2.25–2.75 mmol/L
3–12 y	8.8–10.8 mg/dL	2.20–2.70 mmol/L
13–18 y	8.4–10.2 mg/dL	2.10–2.55 mmol/L
Adult	8.2–10.2 mg/dL	2.05–2.55 mmol/L
Adult older than 90 y	8.2–9.6 mg/dL	2.05–2.40 mmol/L

Ca2+ plays a major role in cellular metabolic functions such as muscle and nerve contraction, enzyme release, blood clotting, and cell growth. As a consequence, low plasma [Ca2+] (hypocalcemia), or high plasma [Ca2+] (hypercalcemia), can lead to serious cellular dysfunction.

Ca2+ Homeostasis
Plasma [Ca2+] is preserved under specific limits by the relationship of intestinal, bone, and kidney resorption and production of Ca2+. Thus, the interaction between these three organs retains the plasma Ca2+ level within a limited range. Ca2+ homeostasis is maintained by three hormones and the Ca2+-sensing receptor system:
1. Ca2+-sensing receptor
2. Parathyroid hormone (PTH)
3. Active vitamin D3 (1,25-dihydroxy-chole-calciferol)
4. Calcitonin

Ca2+-Sensing Receptor (CaSR)

The Ca2+-sensing receptor (CaSR) is expressed in the cells' plasma membranes involved in the homeostasis of Ca2+. CaSR is present in bone cells, thyroid, brain, intestines, and other organs, but its expression is highest in parathyroid glands and kidneys.

- In humans, CaSR senses the circulating levels of Ca2+ and translates this information through a complex signaling pathway, to inhibit or stimulate PTH secretion by the main cells of the parathyroid gland. Low serum Ca2+ levels inhibit CaSR so that PTH is secreted, while high Ca2+ levels activate CaSR and reduce PTH secretion.
- In the kidney, activation of CaSR in the thick ascending limb of Henle's loop prevents paracellular transport of Ca2+, resulting in hypercalciuria. CaSR is found in the inner medullary collection duct in endosomes containing the vasopressin-regulated water receptor, aquaporin 2. Activation of CaSR induces a drop in water absorption induced by vasopressin. This results in polyuria, especially hypercalcemia, which prevents the development of nephrocalcinosis and nephrolithiasis.
- CaSR prevents the development and activity of osteoclasts in the bone, and activates osteoblasts.
- In thyroid C cells, activation of CaSR by high serum Ca2+ induces calcitonin's secretion and facilitates bone formation by taking Ca2+.

PTH

The parathyroid gland secretes PTH. PTH secretion is mainly regulated by extracellular ionized Ca2+. As little as a 10% rise, or decrease, in plasma [Ca2+] prevents or activates PTH's secretion. This PTH response to changes in Ca2+ is mediated, as mentioned earlier, by CaSR. Some PTH secretion modulators include Calcitriol and Mg2+. Calcitriol and hypomagnesemia inhibit the secretion and synthesis of PTH.

PTH manages the plasma [Ca2+] by three mechanisms:

(1) promotes bone resorption (demineralization) by stimulating osteoclasts (cells that break down bone minerals)

(2) improves the synthesis of Calcitriol by improving the activity of 25-hydroxycholecalciferol-1α-hydroxylase (1, α-hydroxylase).

(3) it increases Ca2+ reabsorption in the distal convoluted tubule. Calcitriol increases bone resorption in concert with PTH and also promotes Ca2+ absorption from the intestine.

Active Vitamin D3 (1,25-Dihydroxycholecalciferol, or 1,25(OH)2D3, or Calcitriol)

As stated earlier, Calcitriol is an active form of vitamin D3. It is formed from 25-dihydroxyvitamin D (25(OH)D3) by the enzyme 1, α-hydroxylase, in the proximal tubule cells. PTH stimulates the activity of 1, α-hydroxylase, whereas hypercalcemia and hyperphosphatemia inhibit this enzyme. In the intestine, Calcitriol promotes Ca2+ absorption.

Active vitamin D3 regulates Ca2+ metabolism by four mechanisms:

(1) it stimulates renal Ca2+ reabsorption in distal convoluted tubules
(2) it increases intestinal absorption of Ca2+
(3) it increases the release of Ca2+ from the bone (resorption).
(4) it inhibits PTH synthesis independent of serum [Ca2+].

Certain physiological conditions influence the intestinal absorption of Ca2+.

Normal pregnancy and growth are associated with increased absorption, whereas aging causes decreased absorption. Foods containing oxalates and phytates also decrease intestinal absorption of Ca2+.

Calcitonin

Calcitonin is synthesized by the parafollicular or C cells of the thyroid gland. It is released in response to elevated plasma [Ca2+]. Calcitonin inhibits bone resorption directly by inhibiting osteoclasts' activity and maintaining the plasma [Ca2+] within narrow limits.

Renal Handling of Ca2+

Only ionized and anion-complexed Ca2+ can be filtered. The proximal tubule reabsorbs approximately 65% of the filtered Ca2+, 25% by the thick ascending limb of Henle's loop, 5–10% by the distal convoluted tubule, and 5% by the collecting duct. Less than 2% of Ca2+ is excreted in the urine.

Proximal Tubule

In the proximal tubule, Ca2+ reabsorption is mostly passive in conjunction with Na+ and water reabsorption. Na+ and water reabsorption create a concentration gradient that drives Ca2+ via the paracellular pathway.

Thick Ascending Limb

In Henle's loop, especially in the thick ascending limb, the lumen is electropositive due to Na/K/2Cl co-transporter activity and back-leak of K+ via ROMK. This causes Ca2+ to diffuse passively via the paracellular pathway into the blood.

Distal and Connecting Tubule

In the distal convoluted and connecting tubules, Ca2+ transport is an active process and therefore occurs against an electrochemical gradient. These segments are the major regulatory sites for Ca2+ excretion in the urine. Ca2+ enters the cell, through the apical transient receptor potential vanilloid 5 (TRPV5) Ca2+ channel.

Collecting Duct

Ca2+ transport in the collecting duct is minor compared to the other segments of the nephron. The transport may be active in the cortical collecting duct and passive in the medullary segment.

Factors Influencing Ca2+ Transport

Several factors either decrease or increase Ca2+ reabsorption in various segments of the nephron. As a result, the urinary excretion of Ca2+ varies.

- PTH is an important regulator. It promotes Ca2+ reabsorption by the thick ascending limb of Henle's loop and the distal convoluted tubule, but its effects on the proximal tubule are variable (increase, decrease, or no effect).
- Calcitonin also has variable effects.
- Vitamin D may stimulate Ca2+ reabsorption in the distal convoluted tubule by stimulating the production of Ca2+-binding proteins (calbindins).
- Hypercalcemia decreases Ca2+ reabsorption via a decrease in PTH secretion and enhances Ca2+ excretion.

- Volume expansion reduces Ca2+ reabsorption, whereas volume contraction promotes Ca2+ reabsorption.
- Metabolic acidosis inhibits Ca2+ reabsorption in the proximal and distal convoluted tubule and promotes Ca2+ excretion. Metabolic alkalosis has the opposite effect.
- Diuretics influence Ca2+ reabsorption and its excretion.
- Loop diuretics, for example, furosemide, and bumetanide, inhibit Ca2+ reabsorption in Henle's loop's thick ascending limb, thereby promoting Ca2+ excretion.
- Acute administration of thiazides promotes Ca2+ reabsorption in the distal convoluted tubule. The urinary excretion of Ca2+ may transiently increase due to marked natriuresis.
- Conversely, thiazides' chronic administration causes hypocalciuria due to enhanced Ca2+ reabsorption in the proximal tubule, caused by volume contraction.
- Amiloride also promotes Ca2+ reabsorption in the distal convoluted tubule.

Factors Influencing Ca2+ Channel (TRPV5)
Studies have shown that several factors influence TRPV5, resulting in changes in Ca2+ reabsorption in the distal convoluted and connecting tubule.

Hypocalcemia

The interrelationship maintains $Ca2+$ homeostasis between intestinal absorption, bone turnover, and renal excretion. Changes in either of these functions can lead to changes in the extracellular $[Ca2+]$. Hypocalcemia is defined in the plasma $[Ca2+] < 8.5$ mg/dL. Hypocalcemia is less common than hypercalcemia; because $Ca2+$ is bound to albumin, a decrease in plasma albumin concentration can induce hypocalcemia. For each gram of albumin decrease from normal (i.e. 4.0 g/dL), $[Ca2+]$ decreases by 0.8 mg/dL.

Causes of Hypocalcemia

Pseudohypocalcemia

- MRI with contrast agents (gadodiamide and gadoversetamide) interferes with colorimetric determination of $Ca2+$
- Low serum albumin levels (for each gram decrease in serum albumin from 4.0 g/dL, serum $Ca2+$ decreases by 0.8 mg/dL)
- Decreased synthesis (poor intake, liver disease, infection, or inflammation)
- Nephrotic syndrome
- Protein-losing enteropathy.

Low or absent parathyroid hormone (PTH) levels
Hypoparathyroidism

Genetic

- Parathyroid agenesis. Branchial dysembryogenesis (DiGeorge's syndrome)
- Autoimmune. Polyglandular autoimmune disorder type 1
- Activating mutations of CaSR, an autosomal dominant disorder characterized by hypocalcemia, low PTH levels, neonatal seizures, and carpopedal spasm.

Acquired

- Parathyroid destruction. Parathyroid surgery, infiltrative diseases, irradiation
- Hypomagnesemia. Inhibition of PTH secretion and/or PTH resistance to bone resorption
- Neonatal Hypocalcemia. Functional maternal hypoparathyroidism; maternal hypercalcemia with suppression of PTH levels.

High PTH levels

Pseudo-hypoparathyroidism. Resistance to PTH action

- Disturbance in vitamin D metabolism
- Decreased oral intake. Malnutrition
- Decreased intestinal absorption. Gastrectomy, intestinal by-pass
- Decreased production of 25(OH)D3. Liver disease
- Decreased synthesis of 1,25(OH)2D3. Renal failure, hyper-phosphatemia (inhibits 1α-hydroxylase)
- Increased urinary loss of 25(OH)D3. Nephrotic syndrome.

Drugs

- Anticonvulsants. Increased metabolism of 25(OH)D3, decreased Ca^{2+} release from bone, decreased intestinal absorption of Ca^{2+}
- Bisphosphonates inhibit bone resorption ($\downarrow$ osteoclast activity)
- Denosumab inhibits bone resorption
- Calcitonin inhibits bone resorption
- Citrate. Chelates Ca^{2+}
- Foscarnet, fluoride. Chelate Ca^{2+}
- Antibiotics. Hypocalcemia (a consequence of hypomagnesemia)
- Cinacalcet. Inhibition of PTH secretion by activation of CaSR
- Phosphate binders (calcium acetate). Bind phosphate in the gut and decrease Ca^{2+} absorption

<u>Miscellaneous</u>

- Pancreatitis due to Ca^{2+} deposition at sites of fat necrosis as Ca^{2+} soaps, relative hypoparathyroidism, high glucagon levels, hypomagnesemia, and shift of Ca^{2+} from extracellular to the intracellular compartment by catecholamines
- Sepsis and toxic shock syndrome. The exact mechanism unknown (TNF, IL-2 may mediate)
- "Hungry bone syndrome" because of Ca^{2+} uptake by bones following parathyroid surgery
- Increased osteoblastic activity, as hypocalcemia seen in breast and prostate cancer is due to consumption for bone formation, and due to increased metastatic osteoblast activity
- Chronic respiratory alkalosis, or metabolic alkalosis

- Binding of Ca2+ to albumin, resulting in hypocalcemia
- Rhabdomyolysis or tumor lysis syndrome. Hyperphosphatemia-induced hypocalcemia.

Reasons for Hypocalcemia
Bear in mind: "**Low Calcium**"
Low parathyroid hormone due to the destruction or removal of the parathyroid gland (after any neck ex: thyroidectomy surgeries, you want to check the calcium level).
Oral intake is not adequate (bulimia, alcoholism, etc.)
Wound drainage (particularly GI System because this is where calcium is absorbed)
Celiac & Crohn's Disease trigger malabsorption of calcium in the GI tract.
Acute Pancreatitis.
Low/reduced Vitamin D concentrations (permits for calcium to be resorbed).
Chronic kidney issues (disproportionate excretion of calcium through the kidneys).
Increased phosphorus levels in the blood (phosphorus and calcium do the opposite of each other).
Using medications such as magnesium supplements, laxatives, loop diuretics, calcium binder drugs.
Mobility issues.

Diagnosis
Step 1
• Obtain surgical history and good history regarding nutrition, medications, and inherited and developmental anomalies.
• Physical examination should focus on blood pressure (usually hypotension), bradycardia, and neurologic and ocular (cataracts) changes.
Step 2
• Rule out pseudohypocalcemia following magnetic resonance imaging (MRI) with contrast agents.
Step 3
• Establish true hypocalcemia by determining serum ionized Ca^{2+}.
Step 4
• Determine serum albumin and correct Ca^{2+} for normal albumin concentration.
Step 5
• Measure serum Mg^{2+} and phosphate. Correct hypomagnesemia and hyperphosphatemia.
Step 6
• Review medications that alter 25(OH)D3 (calcifediol) metabolism and change or choose alternative medications.
Step 7
• Check liver and renal functions.
Step 8
• Determine serum PTH and vitamin D status. Start vitamin D preparations for vitamin D deficiency.
Step 9
• If PTH is elevated, evaluate parathyroid glands. If PTH resistance is suspected, measure urinary cAMP levels in response to PTH infusion.

Clinical manifestations of hypocalcemia

The clinical manifestations hinge on the severity of hypocalcemia and the duration of its onset. Also, associated conditions such as alkaline pH, hypomagnesemia, and hypokalemia may precipitate the sudden onset of hypocalcemia signs and symptoms. Usually, the symptoms are related to neuromuscular, cardiac, and central nervous systems.

Neuromuscular

- Muscle weakness and fatigue

- Perioral, finger, and toe tingling

- Chvostek's sign (tapping over facial nerve next to ear elicits tetany or facial twitching)

- Trousseau's sign (carpopedal spasm: inflation of blood pressure cuff to 20 mm Hg above systolic pressure for 3 min elicits flexion of the wrist, thumb, and metacarpo-phalangeal joints with flexion of fingers).

Cardiovascular

- Prolonged QT interval

- Arrhythmias

- Hypotension

- Cardiomyopathy with congestive heart failure.

Central nervous system

- Altered mental status

- Irritability

- Pseudotumor cerebri

- Tonic-clonic seizures

- Vascular calcification of basal ganglia.

Hypocalcemia (C.R.A.M.P.)
Confusion
Reflexes brisk
Arrhythmias (prolonged QT interval and ST interval)
Muscle spasms in calves or feet, seizures, tetany
Positive Trousseaus! You will see this before the sign of Chvostek or before the tetany. This symptom can be positive before other signs of hypocalcemia, such as hyperactive reflexes.

Or

Remember **CATS**
Confusion/Convulsions
Arrhythmias
Tetany
Spasms, stridors, seizures.

Treatment

Acute Hypocalcemia
• Signs and symptoms of acute hypocalcemia usually occur in hospital settings: following thyroid, parathyroid, or neck surgery, during transfusion of citrated blood, and during plasma exchange.
• Injection of calcium gluconate (1 g available as 10% in a 10 mL ampule) is the preferred treatment for symptomatic hypocalcemia for intravenous use.
• Each gram of calcium gluconate contains 93 mg of elemental Ca^{2+}.
• Initially, one to two calcium gluconate ampoules with 5 percent dextrose infusion of 50 mL should be administered over 10–20 min, followed by 0.3–1 mg of elemental Ca^{2+}/kg/h, if necessary. Once symptoms improve, the patient can start using oral Ca^{2+} tablets.

• In order to increase the overall serum Ca2+ by 2–3 mg/dL, a 70 kg patient requires 1 g of elemental Ca2+ (approximately 10 calcium gluconate ampoules).

• One gram of calcium chloride (10 percent) contains 273 mg of elemental Ca2+; however, it is not always preferred to vein due to its intolerable discomfort. However, it can be used to treat acute hypocalcemia in a highly symptomatic condition.

• One gram of *calcium gluceptate* (22% solution in 5 mL ampoule) contains 90 mg of elemental Ca2+.

• If hypomagnesemia is the underlying cause of hypocalcemia, IV magnesium sulfate (8 mEq) should be given.

• Hyperphosphatemia-induced hypocalcemia responds to phosphate binders or hemodialysis.

• For patients immediately following parathyroid surgery owing to primary hyperparathyroidism, or hyperparathyroidism with renal osteodystrophy in chronic kidney disease stage 5, either Calcitriol (Rocaltrol) 1–2 μg orally or IV Calcijex 1–2 μg along with IV calcium supplements may be necessary. Once the patient is stable, any oral vitamin D should be started as indicated.

Chronic Hypocalcemia

- Therapy is meant to remedy the cause, if possible.
- Oral calcium supplements (500–1,500 mg elemental Ca2+) and calcitriol 0.5–1 μg/day are widely used for hypoparathyroidism or PTH resistance, chronic kidney failure, and osteomalacia.
- Certain patients with hypoparathyroidism can benefit from thiazide diuretics.
- Cholecalciferol (effective dose 400–1,000 U/day) or ergocalciferol (effective dose 25,000–50,000 U three times/week) can be used in patients with dietary vitamin D deficiency.
- Aim to maintain serum [Ca2+] slightly below normal to avoid hypercalciuria and subsequent nephrolithiasis.
- Help the intake of calcium-rich food.

Young Sally's Calcium Serum Continues To Randomly Mess-up.
• Yogurt
• Sardines
• Cheese
• Spinach
• Collard greens
• Tofu
• Rhubarb
• Milk

Important to remember:

- Abnormal levels of calcium are used to imply general malfunctions in various body systems. Measurement of ionized calcium is used under more specific conditions.
- Calcium values should be viewed following other test results.
- Normal calcium with a high phosphorus value indicates decreased calcium absorption (possibly due to altered parathyroid hormone levels or activity).
- Normal calcium with an elevated value of urea nitrogen indicates possible hyperparathyroidism (primary or secondary).
- Standard calcium with decreased albumin content is an indicator of hypercalcemia. Hypoalbuminemia is the most frequent cause of hypocalcemia (low calcium levels).
- Hyperparathyroidism and cancer are the most common causes of hypercalcemia (high calcium levels).

Hypercalcemia

Hypercalcemia is defined as serum [Ca2+] >10.2 mg/dL in an individual with normal serum albumin concentration. Generally, severe hypercalcemia is considered when serum [Ca2+] is above 14 mg/dL. Hypercalcemia affects various organs in the body, such as the kidney, heart, brain, peripheral nerves, and intestines.

Causes of Hypercalcemia

Although the causes of hypercalcemia vary, they fall into four main categories:
(1) secondary hypercalcemia due to expanded bone mobilization of Ca2+
(2) hypercalcemia due to increased absorption of Ca2+ from the digestive (GI) tract
(3) hypercalcemia due to reduced urinary excretion of Ca2+
(4) hypercalcemia due to medications.

Hypercalcemia secondary to increased Ca2+ *mobilization from the bone*

- Primary hyperparathyroidism. Increased bone resorption
- Multiple endocrine neoplasias I and 2A
- Pseudo-hypoparathyroidism
- Renal failure
- Secondary hyper-parathyroidism
- Tertiary hyper-parathyroidism
- Acute kidney failure, mostly during the recovery phase
- Malignancy
- Hyperthyroidism
- Immobilization
- Addison's disease. Hemoconcentration, ↑ albumin, bone resorption.

Hypercalcemia due to increased absorption of Ca2+ from the GI tract

- Granulomatous diseases (sarcoidosis, tuberculosis, histoplasmosis, coccidioidomycosis, berylliosis, leprosy, silicone)
- Increased production of calcitriol by elevated 1, α-hydroxylase activity, and increased GI and renal absorption of Ca2+
- Vitamin D intoxication
- Milk (calcium)-alkali syndrome.

Hypercalcemia due to decreased urinary excretion of Ca2+

- Thiazide diuretics. Increased Ca2+ reabsorption by the proximal tubule
- Familial hypercalcemic hypocalciuria. Inactivating mutations of Ca2+-sensing receptor (CaSR).

Medications (other than thiazide diuretics)

- Lithium. Increased PTH secretion
- Vitamin D. Increased GI absorption of Ca2+
- Vitamin A. Increased bone resorption
- Growth hormone. By unknown mechanism
- Estrogens/antiestrogens. Increased bone resorption ↓ sensitivity of parathyroids to Ca2+
- Theophylline β2–agonist mediation.

The mnemonic "CHIMPANZEES can remember causes of hypercalcemia."
• C – Calcium supplementation
• H – Hydrochlorothiazide
• I – Iatrogenic, immobilization
• M – Multiple myeloma, milk-alkali syndrome, medication (e.g. Lithium)
• P – Parathyroid hyperplasia or adenoma
• A – Alcohol

• N – Neoplasm (e.g. breast cancer, lung cancer)
• Z – ZollingerEllison syndrome
• E – Excessive vitamin D
• E – Excessive vitamin A
• S – Sarcoidosis

Clinical Manifestations

Since Ca2+ is essential for the functions of all organs, hypercalcemia affects all organ systems. Signs and signs of hypercalcemia depend on the magnitude and rate of rising in Ca2+ levels. Based on the serum Ca2+ levels, hypercalcemia is graded as mild (10.3–11.9 mg/dL), moderate (12–13.9 mg/dL) and severe (>14 mg/dL) hypercalcemia. Renal and neurological symptoms intensify with elevated hypercalcemia.

Besides, the sudden occurrence of mild to moderate hypercalcemia results in serious neurological dysfunction. Chronic hypercalcemia, on the other hand, may induce minor neurological signs and symptoms. Mild hypercalcemia may be asymptomatic in younger people, but may profoundly impact the elderly due to pre-existing neurological and cognitive dysfunction, general weakness, malaise, and tiredness.

Neuromuscular and psychiatric
Confusion, impaired memory, lethargy, stupor, coma, muscle weakness, and hypotonia.

Cardiac
Short QT interval, arrhythmias, bundle branch blocks, and hypertension.

Renal
Dehydration, polyuria, polydipsia, nocturia (nephrogenic DI), nephrocalcinosis, nephrolithiasis, tubulointerstitial disease, and both acute and chronic kidney disease.

Gastrointestinal
Nausea, vomiting, poor appetite, weight loss, constipation, abdominal pain, and pancreatitis.

Skeletal
Bone pain, arthritis, osteoporosis, osteitis fibrosa cystica.

Calcifications
Band keratopathy, red-eye syndrome, and conjunctival and vascular calcifications.

Hypercalcemia (W.E.A.K.)
• The weakness of muscles (Fewer action potentials)
• EKG changes
• Absent reflexes (Fewer action potentials)
• Kidney Stone Formation

Diagnosis

Step 1
Confirm true hypercalcemia by measuring serum and ionized Ca^{2+} after hemoconcentration; Ca^{2+}-binding paraproteinemia or thrombocythemia-associated hypercalcemia (Ca^{2+} is released from platelets) have been ruled out.

Step 2
Obtain electrolytes, creatinine, BUN, albumin, phosphate, and alkaline phosphatase, as well as complete blood count.

Step 3
History:

- Take a good history regarding signs and symptoms of hypercalcemia and medications.
- Inquire about the shortness of breath and evaluate the most recent chest X-ray as well as electrocardiography (EKG).
- Also, inquire about frequent urination, abdominal pain, and/or constipation.
- History of low back pain, bone pain, ulcer disease, and kidney stones suggest chronic hypercalcemia. Establish acute onset or chronicity of hypercalcemia.

Physical examination
It should include evaluating blood pressure and pulse, volume status, eye examination for calcification, and neurologic status.

Step 4
Intact PTH determination is the single most crucial test in the differential diagnosis of hypercalcemia. Besides, PTHrP and vitamin D levels are usually ordered.

Step 5
Also, 24 h urinary Ca2+ excretion or fractional excretion of Ca2+ can be useful in the differential diagnosis of hypercalcemia.

Step 6
If parathyroidectomy is indicated, a Sestamibi scan can be ordered. If malignancy is suspected, urine and serum immunoelectrophoresis, computed tomography (CT) of the chest and abdomen, and a mammogram should be obtained.

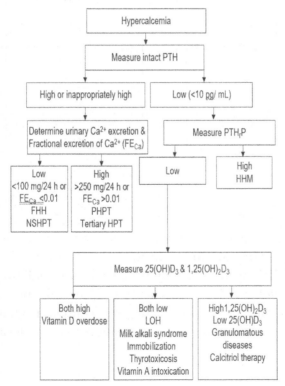

Condition	PO$_4$	PTH	PTHrP	25(OH)D$_3$	1,25(OH)$_2$D$_3$	UCa	UcAMP
Primary hyperparathyroidism	↓	↑	UD	N	↑	↑	↑
Secondary hyperparathyroidism	↑	↑	N	N	↓	NS	NS
FHH	↑	N/↑	UD	N	N	↓	N
Tumor-induced bone resorption	N/↑	↓	N/↑	N	N/↓	N/↑	N/↓
Humoral hypercalcemia of malignancy	N/↓	↓	↑	N	N/↓	↑	↑
Granulomatous diseases	N/↑	↓	UD	N	↑	↑	N
Vitamin D toxicity	N/↑	↓	UD	↑	N/↑/↓	↑	↓
Milk-alkali syndrome	N/↓	↓	UD	↑	↓	↓	N/↓

Treatment

The primary goal of treatment of hypercalcemia is the correction of the underlying cause. For example, parathyroidectomy is the definitive treatment for PHPT. Similarly, chemotherapy for malignant disease improves hypercalcemia. However, acute treatment is indicated in patients with signs and symptoms of hypercalcemia. In general, these signs and symptoms are mostly related to neuropsychiatric and GI systems.

Acute Treatment

The treatment of acute hypercalcemia includes:

1. Hydration with normal saline and then judicious administration of furosemide for volume overload. Note that furosemide-induced volume depletion may increase the reabsorption of Ca2+ by the proximal tubule; many physicians thus doubt furosemide's efficacy in treating acute hypercalcemia.

2. Inhibition of Ca2+ bone resorption.
3. Reduced absorption of Ca2+ through the intestine.
4. Removal of Ca2+ by hemodialysis using a low Ca2+ dialysate bath.

Treatment	Dosage	Route	Duration of effect	Mechanism
Promote Ca²⁺ excretion				
Normal saline	1–2 L every 6 h	IV	4–6 h	Improves GFR and promotes Ca^{2+} excretion
Furosemide	40–120 mg every 2–4 h	IV	2–4 h	Inhibits Ca^{2+} reabsorption in TALH
Decrease bone resorption				
Calcitonin	2–4 MRC units/kg every 4–8 h	IV	4–12 h	Inhibits bone resorption
Pamidronate[a]	30–90 mg in 100–200 mL saline or D5W once	IV over 4–24 h	2–3 weeks	Inhibits bone resorption. Clinical response takes 2–3 days
Zoledronate[a]	4 mg in 50 mL of saline or D5W once	IV over 15–20 min	2–3 weeks	Inhibits bone resorption. Clinical response takes 2–3 days
Gallium citrate	200 mg/m²/day in 1 L of saline for 5 days	IV	1–2 weeks	Inhibits bone resorption
Decrease intestinal absorption				
Prednisone	20–30 mg every 12 h	Oral	2–4 days	Inhibits gut absorption
Decrease plasma [Ca²⁺]				
Hemodialysis	Use dialysate bath containing low Ca^{2+}		Few hours	Removal from blood

Chronic Treatment

Chronic management of hypercalcemia includes the removal of the cause.

The goals of therapy include:

1. Fixed root cause: parathyroidectomy and chemotherapy. Consider cinacalcet (30-120 mg/day) for secondary hyperparathyroidism. Judiciary use of cinacalcet in individual patients with PHPT is recommended.

2. Maintenance of euvolemia: prescribe an adequate amount of water equal to or slightly more than urine output and insensible loss.

3. Decrease in the synthesis of 1,25(OH)2D3: low calcium diet, reduce vitamin D intake, hormones, chloroquine (250 mg/day), hydroxychloroquine (400–600 mg/day), and ketoconazole (100–200 mg/day).

4. Decrease intestinal absorption of Ca2+: low calcium diet, steroids, and the avoidance of vitamin D supplements.
5. Decrease in bone resorption: steroids, lower PTH levels, reduce vitamin D use, bisphosphonates, and nuclear factor-kB ligand (RANKL) enzyme receptor activator, and denosumab.
6. Bisphosphonates are used for the prevention of hypercalcemia in patients with malignancy. They prevent bone resorption caused by osteoclasts. Only pamidronate and zoledronate are approved for acute hypercalcemia management of malignancy in the USA, out of the available bisphosphonates. Ibandronate is approved in Europe. All are excreted through urine. Reduction in the dose and slow infusion are recommended in patients with renal failure. Zoledronate is more potent than pamidronate. The effect of bisphosphonates is seen in 48–72 h and lasts for 2–3 weeks. Repeat the dose, if necessary.

7. Denosumab is a humanized monoclonal antibody that impedes osteoclastic activity and, therefore, bone resorption. It was initially approved for postmenopausal women with osteoporosis. It reduces serum Ca2+ level. Subsequently, it was approved for skeletal-related events such as hypercalcemia in patients with bone metastasis due to a solid tumor. Thus, denosumab is recommended for tumor-induced hypercalcemia when bisphosphonates do not work, or failed to work.

Chapter 6
Serum Phosphate

Phosphate comprises approximately 1% of the body weight. In plasma, phosphate exists in two forms, *organic* (70%) and *inorganic* (30%). Phosphate plays a significant role in mitochondrial respiration and oxidative phosphorylation. In plasma, phosphorus concentration is stated as mg/dL, and in transport and other processes, it is usually expressed as mEq or mmol/L.

Age	Conventional Units	SI Units (Conversion Factor 0.323)
0–5 days	4.6–8.0 mg/dL	1.5–2.6 mmol/L
1–3 years	3.9–6.5 mg/dL	1.3–2.1 mmol/L
4–6 years	4.0–5.4 mg/dL	1.3–1.7 mmol/L
7–11 years	3.7–5.6 mg/dL	1.2–1.8 mmol/L
12–13 years	3.3–5.4 mg/dL	1.1–1.7 mmol/L
14–15 years	2.9–5.4 mg/dL	0.9–1.7 mmol/L
16–19 years	2.8–4.6 mg/dL	0.9–1.5 mmol/L
>19 years	2.5–4.5 mg/dL	0.8–1.4 mmol/L

Inorganic forms are physiologically active. Just 10% of inorganic phosphate is attached to albumin. However, unlike $Ca2+$, phosphate concentration is not impaired by changes in the concentration of plasma albumin. The concentration of intracellular phosphate is several times greater than the plasma concentration. Within the cell, 75% of phosphate occurs as organic phosphate compounds such as adenosine triphosphate (ATP), creatine phosphate, and adenosine monophosphate. It exists mainly as 2,3-diphosphoglycerate in red blood cells. Free phosphate in the cytosol accounts for 25% of the phosphate's intracellular concentration, and only this fraction is available for transport mechanisms.

Phosphate Homeostasis

As in Ca2+ homeostasis, three main organs are involved in phosphate homeostasis: the intestine, the kidney, and the bone. When the phosphate's gut absorption increases, a transient increase in plasma [Pi] occurs, and the kidneys excrete this excess amount to maintain the normal plasma [Pi].

In the intestine, both absorption and secretion of phosphate occur. Most of the dietary phosphate is absorbed in the duodenum and jejunum. Some phosphate is also secreted into saliva and bile. Under normal conditions, the exchange of phosphate between the bone and the extracellular pool is relatively small, and the release of Ca2+ always accompanies the release of phosphate. Thus, the release of phosphate is stimulated by the same hormones that stimulate the release of Ca2+.

The kidneys play a considerable role in the maintenance of phosphate homeostasis. Since phosphate's dietary intake varies daily, the total body phosphate concentration would also vary, were it not for the kidneys. The kidneys vary their phosphate excretion to the varying amounts of phosphate absorption by the intestine, to maintain normal serum [Pi].

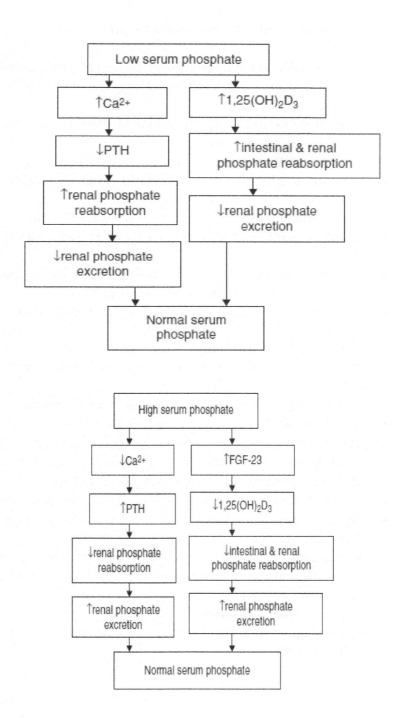

The factors that control Phosphate homeostasis

Factors that inhibit phosphate reabsorption and increase excretion
- PTH Inhibition of Na/Pi-IIa and IIc co-transport and Na/K-ATPase
- FGF-23 Inhibition of type IIa and decreased formation of calcitriol by 1,α-hydroxylase inhibition
- Calcitriol. Inhibition of type IIa co-transporter
- Dopamine. Inhibition of type IIa co-transporter and Na/K-ATPase
- Glucocorticoids. Inhibition of type IIa co-transporter
- Volume expansion. Increase in GFR and reduced Na+ reabsorption
- Chronic metabolic acidosis. Inhibition of type IIa co-transporter and resorption of phosphate from bone
- High phosphate intake. Inhibition of type IIa and IIc co-transporters
- Diuretics. Probably related to decreased Na+ reabsorptions. Also, carbonic anhydrase inhibitors decrease type IIa co-transporter
- Chronic hypercalcemia. Through unknown mechanism
- Hypokalemia. Inhibition of type IIc co-transporter.

Factors that promote phosphate reabsorption and decrease excretion
- Parathyroidectomy. Increased type IIa co-transporter activity
- Insulin. Increased type IIa co-transporter activity
- Growth hormone. Increased type IIa co-transporter activity
- Volume contraction. Decreased GFR associated with increased Na+ reabsorption
- Metabolic alkalosis. Increased type IIa co-transporter activity
- Low phosphate intake. Increased type IIa and type IIc co-transporter activity
- Hypocalcemia. Unknown
- Hypermagnesemia. Increased type IIa and type IIc co-transporter activity.

Hypophosphatemia

Hypophosphatemia is characterised as serum [Pi] <2.5 mg/dL. Hypophosphatemia can be severe (blood [Pi] <1.0 mg/dL), moderate (serum [Pi] 1.0–1.9 mg/dL) or mild (serum [Pi] 2.0–2.5 mg/dL). Extreme hypophosphatemia can occur in patients with repeated antacids such as aluminum hydroxide, magnesium hydroxide, or calcium carbonate or acetate. Moderate hypophosphatemia could be symptomatic or asymptomatic. Hypophosphatemia is relatively uncommon in the common population. However, hypophosphatemia in hospitalized patients with sepsis, chronic alcoholism, and chronic obstructive pulmonary disease (COPD) is high. Patients with trauma also have a high incidence of hypophosphatemia.

Causes of Hypophosphatemia
The causes are varied, but can be grouped simply under four categories:

Shift from extracellular to the intracellular compartment
- Glucose. Transcellular distribution
- Insulin. Transcellular distribution
- Catecholamines. Transcellular distribution
- Hyperalimentation. Glucose-induced cellular uptake
- Respiratory alkalosis. Transcellular distribution
- Refeeding syndrome. Glucose and insulin-induced transcellular distribution, consumption during glucose metabolism, and ATP production
- Rapid cellular proliferation. Cellular uptake.

Decreased intestinal absorption
- Poor dietary intake/starvation ↓ intestinal absorption
- Malabsorption. Disorders of duodenum and jejunum (celiac disease, tropical and nontropical sprue, regional enteritis), ↓ intestinal absorption
- Phosphate binders. Calcium acetate or bicarbonate, aluminum hydroxide, and magnesium salts bind phosphate in the gut
- Vitamin deficiency ↓ intestinal absorption
- Vitamin D-dependent (VDD) rickets
- Type I VDD rickets. Low or deficiency of $1,25(OH)_2D_3$

- Type 2 VDD rickets. Resistance to 1,25(OH)2D3 action.

Increased renal loss

- Primary and secondary hyperparathyroidism ↓ renal absorption
- Increased fibroblast growth factor (FGF)-23 production or activity ↓ renal absorption.

Inherited disorders

- X-linked hypophosphatemia. Mutations in the PHEX gene
- Autosomal dominant hypophosphatemia
- Mutations in FGF-23 gene
- Autosomal recessive hypophosphatemia
- Mutations in DMP1 and ENPP1 genes.

Acquired disorders

- Tumor-induced osteomalacia. Increased FGF-23 secretion and activity
- Proximal tubule defect in phosphate reabsorption ↓ renal absorption
- Hereditary hypophosphatemic rickets with hypercalciuria
- Mutations in the gene-encoding Na/Pi-IIc co-transporter
- Autosomal recessive renal phosphate-wasting
- Mutations in the gene-encoding Na/Pi-IIa co-transporter
- Fanconi syndrome. A disorder causing decreased reabsorption of glucose, phosphate, amino acids, uric acid, bicarbonate, calcium, and potassium. Can be genetic or acquired
- Renal transplantation. Tertiary hyperparathyroidism, excess FGF-23, immunosuppressive drugs, low 25(OH)D3 and 1,25(OH)2D3 levels
- Volume expansion, post-obstructive diuresis, hepatectomy ↓ renal reabsorption, and phosphaturia
- Osmotic diuretics ↓ renal reabsorption and phosphaturia
- Carbonic anhydrase inhibitor ↓ renal reabsorption and phosphaturia
- Loop diuretics ↓ renal reabsorption and phosphaturia
- Metolazone ↓ renal reabsorption and phosphaturia
- Acyclovir Inhibition of Na/Pi-IIa co-transporter
- Acetaminophen poisoning ↓ renal reabsorption and phosphaturia

- Intravenous iron administration. Increase in FGF-23 secretion and activity by inhibiting 1, α-hydroxylase
- Tyrosine kinase inhibitors (imatinib, sorafenib) ↓Ca2 + and phosphate reabsorption and secondary hyperparathyroidism
- Corticosteroids ↓ intestinal phosphate absorption and phosphaturia
- Bisphosphonates. Inhibition of bone resorption
- Cyclophosphamide, cisplatin ↑ phosphaturia
- Ifosfamide, streptozotocin, suramin. Induction of Fanconi syndrome
- Aminoglycosides, tetracyclines Induction of Fanconi syndrome
- Valproic acid. Induction of Fanconi syndrome
- Tenofovir, cidofovir, adefovir. Induction of Fanconi syndrome.

Miscellaneous causes
- Alcoholism. Poor intake, frequent use of phosphate binders, vitamin D deficiency, respiratory alkalosis, proximal tubule defect, ↓ intestinal absorption
- Diabetic ketoacidosis ↓ total body phosphate due to osmotic diuresis at onset, and hypophosphatemia after insulin administration
- Toxic shock syndrome. Cellular uptake probably due to respiratory alkalosis.

Patients receiving mannitol may experience pseudohypophosphatemia caused by mannitol binding to the molybdate used to determine the serum [Pi].

Clinical Manifestations

The clinical manifestations of hypophosphatemia depend on its onset and severity. Two biochemical abnormalities underlie the manifestations of phosphate deficiency. One is the depletion of ATP, and the second is a reduction in erythrocyte 2,3-diphosphoglycerate. Both depletions lead to altered cellular function and hypoxia. The following are manifestations of severe hypophosphatemia:

Neurologic
- Confusion
- Irritability
- Anorexia
- Ataxia
- Dysarthria
- Paresthesia
- Seizures
- Coma

Cardiovascular
- Cardiomyopathy
- Decreased cardiac output
- Altered membrane potential

Skeletal muscle
- Muscle weakness
- Rhabdomyolysis
- Bone pain
- Rickets
- Osteomalacia
- Pseudofractures
- Osteopenia

Hematologic
Red blood cells
- Decreased 2,3-diphosphoglycerate content
- Decreased ATP production
- Increased oxygen affinity
- Hemolysis
- Decreased life span

Leukocytes
- Impaired phagocytosis
- Impaired bactericidal activity
- Impaired chemotaxis

Platelets
- Thrombocytopenia

- Decreased life span
- Megakaryocytosis

Carbohydrate metabolism
- Decreased glucose metabolism
- Insulin resistance

Biochemical
- Increased creatine kinase
- Increased aldolase
- Decreased parathyroid hormone (PTH)
- Hypomagnesemia

Renal
- Decreased glomerular filtration rate (GFR)
- Hypercalciuria
- Hypermagnesuria
- Hypophosphaturia
- Increased 1,25(OH)2D3
- Decreased renal gluconeogenesis
- Decreased renal HCO3– threshold
- Decreased net titratable acidity

Respiratory
- Respiratory muscle weakness
- Impaired diaphragmatic contractility
- Respiratory failure
- Difficulty in weaning
- Hypoxia

Diagnosis

Step 1

• First, the cause of hypophosphatemia should be established from the history, physical examination, and the clinical setting in which it occurs.

• History: inquire about signs and symptoms. History of alcoholism and medications is important. In hospitalized patients, a review of dietary intake, IV fluids, and diagnosis is also important.

Step 2

• Physical examination should focus on the musculoskeletal system.

• Muscle tenderness and pain—rhabdomyolysis.

• Pathologic or pseudofractures and skeletal deformities—rickets in children.

• Rachitic features in adults—chronic hypophosphatemia.

• Short stature with increased upper to lower body ratio—previous childhood rickets.

• Sinus tumors—TIO.

• Hepatomegaly—chronic alcoholism, tumors.

• Limited spine, joint, and hip motion in adults—X-linked hypophosphatemia.

Step 3

• Serum electrolytes, Ca2+, phosphate, Mg2+, alkaline phosphatase, and GFR.

• Measure urine phosphate and creatinine.

• Calculate fractional excretion of phosphate (FEPO4), which suggests renal or nonrenal loss of phosphate.

• If FEPO4 is <5%, hypophosphatemia is nonrenal, suggesting transcellular distribution or decreased gastrointestinal absorption.

• If FEPO4 is >5%, hypophosphatemia is renal in origin.

Step 4

• Serum and urine Ca2+, PTH, 25(OH)D3, and 1,25(OH)2D3 levels are usually helpful in the differential diagnosis of various causes of hypophosphatemia.

Step 5

• Increased alkaline phosphatase and PTH levels suggest primary and secondary hyperparathyroidism as well as FGF-23-mediated hypophosphatemia.

• Serum FGF-23 levels are elevated in X-linked hypophosphatemia, ADHR, ARHR, TIO, and after transplantation.

Step 6

• Imaging studies for chronic hypophosphatemia:

– Plain radiographs—fractures and skeletal abnormalities

– Dual-energy X-ray absorptiometry scan—bone density and osteomalacia

– Bone scan—increased uptake of Technetium-99m at multiple sites in osteomalacia

– Computed tomography (CT), magnetic resonance imaging (MRI), positron emission tomography (PET)—TIO.

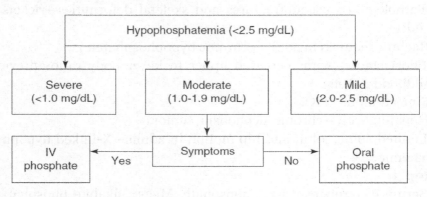

Treatment

Treatment of hypophosphatemia depends on the onset and severity of symptoms, and aims to remove the causes, such as medications or dietary deficiency, whenever possible.

Acute Severe Symptomatic Hypophosphatemia

• It usually occurs in hospitalized patients and carries high morbidity and mortality.

• Although the oral route is the safest, IV administration of either sodium or potassium phosphate with frequent monitoring of serum [Pi] is warranted.

• IV and oral phosphate preparations are as follows:

Treatment	Dosage	Route	Duration of effect	Mechanism
Promote Ca²⁺ excretion				
Normal saline	1–2 L every 6 h	IV	4–6 h	Improves GFR and promotes Ca²⁺ excretion
Furosemide	40–120 mg every 2–4 h	IV	2–4 h	Inhibits Ca²⁺ reabsorption in TALH
Decrease bone resorption				
Calcitonin	2–4 MRC units/kg every 4–8 h	IV	4–12 h	Inhibits bone resorption
Pamidronate[a]	30–90 mg in 100–200 mL saline or D5W once	IV over 4–24 h	2–3 weeks	Inhibits bone resorption. Clinical response takes 2–3 days
Zoledronate[a]	4 mg in 50 mL of saline or D5W once	IV over 15–20 min	2–3 weeks	Inhibits bone resorption. Clinical response takes 2–3 days
Gallium citrate	200 mg/m²/day in 1 L of saline for 5 days	IV	1–2 weeks	Inhibits bone resorption
Decrease intestinal absorption				
Prednisone	20–30 mg every 12 h	Oral	2–4 days	Inhibits gut absorption
Decrease plasma [Ca²⁺]				
Hemodialysis	Use dialysate bath containing low Ca²⁺		Few hours	Removal from blood

• In hyperalimentation-induced hypophosphatemic (< 1.5 mg/dL) patients in an intensive care setting, infusion of 1 mmol/kg (1 mmol = 3.1 mg/dL) phosphorus diluted in 100 or 250 mL of either normal saline or 5% dextrose in water (D5W), at a rate not exceeding 7.5 mmol/h, is sufficient to normalize serum phosphate in 48 h.

• In surgical intensive care patients, a weight-based and serum phosphate-based protocol for IV phosphate repletion is followed. Either sodium or potassium phosphate, depending on serum K+ levels, was dissolved in 250 mL of D5W and infused over 6h as a single dose to severely hypophosphatemic (< 1 mg/dL) or moderately hypophosphatemic (1.5–1.8 mg/dL) patients. Successful repletion occurred in 63% of severe and 78% of moderate hypophosphatemic patients. Thus, severe hypophosphatemic patients may benefit from more aggressive and tailored IV phosphorous regimens.

• Note that IV phosphate administration is associated with hypocalcemia and hyperphosphatemia. Fluid overload in congestive heart failure patients is a problem. In general, moderate hypophosphatemia does not require IV phosphate administration, except when symptoms warrant IV therapy.

• Parenteral calcium is needed in those with combined hypophosphatemia and hypocalcemia. In such cases, *do not* add either bicarbonate or phosphate to calcium-containing solutions.

Serum phosphate	Weight (40–60 kg)	Weight (61–80 kg)	Weight (81–120 kg)
< 0.32 mmol/L (< 1 mg/dL)	30	40	50
0.32–0.54 mmol/L (1–1.7 mg/dL)	20	30	40
0.58–0.7 mmol/L (1.8–2.2 mg/dL)	10	15	20

Chronic Hypophosphatemia
• Management depends on the underlying cause.
• Oral therapy is indicated.

Hyperphosphatemia

Hyperphosphatemia is described as serum [Pi] >4.5 mg/dL.
The causes of true hyperphosphatemia can be discussed under three major categories:
(1) the addition of intracellular fluid (ICF) phosphate to the extracellular fluid (ECF) compartment.
(2) the decline in renal phosphate excretion
(3) drugs.

Major causes of hyperphosphatemia
Acute and chronic kidney failure is perhaps the essential cause of hyperphosphatemia in clinical practice.

Addition of phosphate to extracellular fluid ECF part
Endogenous:
- Hemolysis as phosphate is released from hemolyzed red blood cells
- Rhabdomyolysis as phosphate is released from muscle cells
- In Tumor lysis syndrome, phosphorus is released from tumor cells due to chemotherapy or cell turnover
- High catabolic state leading to release from body cells.

Exogenous:
- Oral intake, or through IV route. Ingestion of sodium phosphate solution for bowel preparation or IV Na/K phosphate in hospitalized patients
- Phosphate-containing enemas. Cause phosphate absorption of enemas (fleet enema) through the gut
- In Respiratory acidosis, phosphate is discharged from the cell
- Lactic acidosis uses phosphate during glycolysis, contributing to its degradation and eventual release from cells
- Diabetic ketoacidosis. Phosphate change from ICF to ECF due to insulin deficiency and metabolic acidosis.

Decreased renal excretion:
- Chronic kidney failure stage 4 and 5. Tendency of the kidneys to excrete phosphate load decreases
- Acute kidney damage. Failure to excrete and release phosphate from muscle during rhabdomyolysis
- Hypoparathyroidism. Enhanced resorption of renal phosphate

- Pseudo-hypoparathyroidism. Renal and skeletal PTH resistance
- Generation of tumor calcinosis due to the mutations in GALNT3, FGF-23, and KLOTHO genes.

Drugs:
- Vitamin D. Improves gastrointestinal (GI) absorption of phosphate
- Bisphosphonates. Cause decreased phosphate excretion, cellular shift
- Growth hormone. Increased proximal tubule reabsorption
- Liposomal amphotericin B. Contains phosphatidylcholine and phosphatidylserine
- Sodium phosphate (oral). GI absorption of phosphate.

A spurious increase in serum [Pi] is called pseudo-hyperphosphatemia. It is relatively rare but has been described in conditions of hyper-globulinemia, hyper-triglyceridemia, and hyper-bilirubinemia. This spurious increase has been attributed to the interference of proteins and triglycerides in phosphate's colorimetric assay.

Clinical Manifestations

Medical symptoms are linked to hypocalcemia-induced hyperphosphatemia (paresthesia, tetanus). In patients with stage 5 CKD and patients on dialysis, hyperphosphatemia and calcium phosphate precipitation are frequent in vascular and muscular systems. Skin deposition is expected as well. Hyperphosphatemia is an autonomous risk factor for all-cause or cardiovascular death in stages 4 and 5 of CKD.

Diagnosis

Step 1

Following the history and physical inspection, full metabolic panels, hemoglobin, and iron indices are obtained. Get PTH and 1,25(OH)2D3 levels.

Step 2

Confirm true hyperphosphatemia only after the elimination of pseudo-hyperphosphatemia.

Step 3

Establish the severity and onset of hyperphosphatemia.

Step 4

Test for blood urea nitrogen (BUN) and creatinine. If normal, look for acute phosphate load (exogenous or endogenous) and those that facilitate renal phosphate reabsorption. If BUN and creatinine are raised, distinguish between AKI and CKD.

Treatment
Hyperphosphatemia is a risk factor for cardiovascular morbidity and mortality, vascular classification, and secondary hyper-parathyroidism. Therefore, control of hyperphosphatemia is significant. The treatment strategies include control of dietary phosphate, phosphate binders, and dialysis.

Diet
The best practice in treating hyperphosphatemia in CKD stage 4 and 5 or dialysis patients is the restriction of dietary proteins and the prevention of phosphate-containing foods. A Dietician's consultation is needed for the prescription of an appropriate diet to prevent malnutrition. Processed foods and beverages that contain phosphate should be minimized in planning a diet for CKD patients. However, owing to poor palatability, patients do not stick to the diet. Regulation of hyperphosphatemia with intestinal phosphate-binding agents is also essential.

Phosphate Binders
The classification of available phosphate binders is as follows:
• Aluminum hydroxide has traditionally been used as a phosphate binder. However, adynamic bone-disease-induced bone pain and fractures, microcytic anemia, and dementia have been reported in many patients. Its use has therefore been discontinued.
• Subsequently, calcium (Ca)-containing binders, such as Ca -carbonate (Caltrate, Os-Cal) and *Ca-acetate* (PhosLo), became available. Although they reduce serum phosphate levels, it became apparent that they cause hypercalcemia and vascular calcification. These complications prompted the nephrologists to use non-Ca-containing binders such as Sevelamer HCl.

• *Sevelamer HCl (Renagel) has been shown to regulate as much phosphate as Ca-containing binders without inducing hypercalcemia.* Studies have also shown that sevelamer slowed coronary artery calcification progression compared with a Ca-containing binder. Besides, sevelamer lowered low-density lipoprotein (LDL) cholesterol levels in dialysis patients, and survival benefit was also reported. It is costly, though, and causes hyperchlorinated metabolic acidosis.

The next generation sevelamer composite has been introduced to improve metabolic acidosis. It is known as sevelamer carbonate (Renvela). Sevelamer carbonate has been shown to have a physiological and biochemical profile similar to sevelamer HCl except for a rise in serum HCO_3- at a level of approximately 2 mEq/L.

• Lanthanum carbonate (Fosrenol), which binds phosphate ionically, is another non-Ca-containing phosphate binder. Unlike other binders, lanthanum carbonate's effectiveness as a binder is so high that medicines-burden decreases, enabling the patient to stick to therapy. Several questions have been raised about its long-term protection as part of the aluminum family in the periodic table. However, no adverse reactions have been shown in dialysis patients who have been followed for 6 years. In one analysis, the rate of hypercalcemia was 0.4 percent in the lanthanum group compared to 20.2 percent in the Ca-treated group.

• Two iron-binding agents (sucroferric oxyhydroxide or Velphoro and ferric citrate or Auryxia) have been introduced in recent years. Both drugs seem to lower phosphate as efficiently as sevelamer.

• *Magnesium (Mg) carbonate is less helpful than Ca-containing binder but is less widely used in patients with dialysis due to fear of diarrhea and exacerbation of hypermagnesemia. However, Mg carbonate may enhance vascular calcification. Despite this beneficial effect, the use of Mg carbonate at this time is not recommended.*

The following summarizes phosphate binders' effects on various biochemical parameters relevant to mineral bone disorder in CKD stage 5 (on dialysis) patients.

Acute Hyperphosphatemia

- Eliminate the cause.
- Use phosphate binders as needed.
- Although not recommended for chronic use, aluminum hydroxide controls moderate hyperphosphatemia in hospitalized patients with normal renal function.
- Hemodialysis is often required when hyperphosphatemia is due to rhabdomyolysis or tumor lysis syndrome.

Chronic Hyperphosphatemia

- Often used in patients with stage 5 CKD and on dialysis.
- The dietary restriction on phosphate is essential.
- Restricted intake of milk, milk products, meat, grains, and processed foods is recommended in consultation with a dietician.
- Phosphate binders are needed in almost all patients on dialysis in addition to dietary restriction.
- Select a phosphate binder that is easy to take and low in cost, provides maximum benefit and has low adverse effects. Unfortunately, none of the phosphate binders fulfills all of these criteria.
- Selection between a Ca-containing binder and a non-Ca-containing binder is difficult.
- Advantages of sevelamer HCl or carbonate are prevention and improvement in vascular calcification.
- Advantage of lanthanum is a decrease in pill burden (3–4 tablets/day). Suitable as second-on drug addition.
- Cinacalcet, a calcimimetic, lowers both Ca^{2+} and phosphate in dialysis patients with secondary hyperparathyroidism.
- Note that long-term oral therapy may suppress $1,25(OH)2D3$ levels and raise PTH and FGF-23 levels. To suppress PTH levels, concomitant administration of calcitriol is suggested. In renal transplant patients, an increase in dietary phosphate may improve hypophosphatemia. Oral phosphate therapy may be indicated in severe hypophosphatemia; however, hyperphosphatemia is a major concern. Therefore, cinacalcet may be indicated in some patients with close monitoring.

Chapter 7
Serum Magnesium

Magnesium (Mg2+) is the second most rich intracellular cation in the body besides K+.

Age	Conventional Units	Alternative Units (Conversion Factor X0.8229)	SI Units (Conversion Factor X0.4114)
New-born	1.5–2.2 mg/dL	1.23–1.81 mEq/L	0.62–0.91 mmol/L
Child	1.7–2.1 mg/dL	1.40–1.73 mEq/L	0.70–0.86 mmol/L
Adult	1.6–2.6 mg/dL	1.32–2.14 mEq/L	0.66–1.07 mmol/L

A 70 kg individual has approximately 25 g of Mg2+. About 67% of Mg2+ is present in the bone, 20% in the muscle, and 12% in other tissues, for instance, the liver. Just the free and non-protein linked Mg2+ is filtered at the glomerulus of the nephron. Mg2+ plays a crucial function in cell metabolism. It is involved in the activation of enzymes such as phosphokinase and phosphatase. Mg-ATPase is also active in ATP hydrolysis and the production of energy used in various ion pump operations. Besides, Mg2+ plays a crucial role in the regulation of protein synthesis and cell volume. Due to its pivotal role in cell physiology, Mg2+ deficiency adversely affects multiple cellular functions.

Mg2+ Homeostasis

The serum concentration of Mg2+ (abbreviated as [Mg2+]) is maintained between 1.7 and 2.7 mg/dL (1.4–2.3 mEq/L).

- As in Ca2+ and phosphate homeostasis, Mg2+ homeostasis is regulated by the intestine, bone, and kidneys. Of ingested Mg2+, 30–40% is absorbed by the jejunum and ileum.
- Intestinal absorption of Mg2+ occurs by transcellular and paracellular pathways.
- Active vitamin D3 (1,25(OH)2D3) increases the intestinal absorption of Mg2+, whereas diets rich in Ca2+ and phosphate decrease its absorption.
- Mg2+ homeostasis is also dependent on the exchange between the extracellular pool and the bone. The Mg2+ available in the surface pool of the bone is involved in the homeostatic regulation of extracellular Mg2+.
- The kidney also maintains Mg2+ homeostasis because it regulates the rate of excretion depending on the Mg2+ concentration. Usually, the excretory fraction of Mg2+ is 5%. In states of Mg2+ deficiency, the excretion can be as low as 0.5%. In states of Mg2+ excess or chronic kidney disease, excretion can be as high as 50%.
- Free and non-protein-bound Mg2+ can be filtered at the glomerulus.
- The most important segment for Mg2+ reabsorption in the cortical thick ascending limb of Henle's loop. In this segment, about 40–70% of Mg2+ is reabsorbed.
-

Factors that Alter Renal Handling of Mg2+ in TALH and DCT

Several factors influence the tubular reabsorption of Mg2+ and are summarized as:

- Volume expansion decreases proximal tubular reabsorption of Na+ and water. As a result, the Mg2+ reabsorption is also decreased. Conversely, volume depletion causes an increase in Mg2+ reabsorption.
- Hypermagnesemia inhibits Mg2+ reabsorption, whereas hypomagnesemia causes renal retention of Mg2+.

- Hypercalcemia markedly increases Mg^{2+} excretion by inhibiting reabsorption in the proximal tubule and TALH. Hypocalcemia has the opposite effect.
- Phosphate depletion enhances Mg^{2+} excretion by reducing its absorption in TALH and DCT.
- Acute acidosis seems to inhibit Mg^{2+} reabsorption in TALH and thus enhances its excretion.
- Chronic metabolic acidosis suppresses TRPM6 expression and activity in DCT and enhances Mg^{2+} excretion.
- On the other hand, metabolic alkalosis decreases urinary excretion of Mg^{2+} by enhancing its reabsorption in the proximal straight tubule and DCT.
- Cyclic AMP-mediated hormones such as parathyroid hormone and ADH enhance Mg^{2+} reabsorption in TALH and DCT and decrease urinary excretion.
- Osmotic diuretics, such as mannitol and urea, promote Mg^{2+} excretion by predominantly inhibiting its reabsorption in TALH and, to some extent, in the proximal tubule.
- Loop diuretics, such as furosemide, inhibit Mg^{2+} reabsorption in TALH and cause magnesuria.
- Thiazide diuretics (hydrochlorothiazide) act in DCT and may cause a mild increase in Mg^{2+} excretion.

Hypomagnesemia

Hypomagnesemia is described as serum [Mg2+] <1.7 mg/dL.
The causes of hypomagnesemia are categorized into four main types:
(1) decreased intake of Mg2+,
(2) decreased intestinal absorption,
(3) increased urinary losses,
(4) drugs.
In addition to these factors, the cellular absorption of Mg2+ is caused
by glucose or epinephrine infusion.

Causes of Hypomagnesemia
Decreased intake
- Protein-calorie malnutrition. Poor Mg2+ intake
- Starvation. Poor Mg2+ intake
- Prolonged IV therapy without Mg2+
- Poor Mg2+ intake
- Chronic alcoholism. Possible mechanisms include
(1) inadequate dietary intake,
(2) alcohol-induced renal Mg2+ loss,
(3) diarrhea,
(4) starvation-ketosis-induced renal Mg2+ loss.

Decreased intestinal absorption

- Prolonged nasogastric suction. Removal from saliva and gastric secretions
- Malabsorption (nontropical sprue and steatorrhea) leading to loss from the intestine
- Diarrhea, as there is loss from the intestine
- Intestinal and biliary fistulas cause magnesium loss from stool and urine
- Excessive use of laxatives causes loss from stool due to diarrhea
- Resection of the small intestine. Defective Mg2+ absorption
- Familial hypomagnesemia with secondary hypocalcemia
- Mutation in the intestinal TRPM6 gene.

Enhanced loss through urine

- Inherited TALH disorders cause familial hypomagnesemia, including hypercalciuria and nephrocalcinosis
- CLDN 16 gene mutations (claudin-16 or paracellin-1) for tight junction proteins cause familial hypomagnesemia with hypercalciuria, and nephrocalcinosis with ocular manifestation
- CLDN19 gene mutation (claudin-19) of the tight junction protein
- Disorders of the Ca/Mg-sensing receptor
- Inactivating mutations in the TALH/DCT Ca/Mg-sensing receptor
- Bartter syndrome. Mutations in Na/K/2Cl, ROMK, ClC-Ka/Kb-Barttin
- Inherited disorders of DCT
- Familial hypomagnesemia with secondary hypocalcemia
- Mutations in the TRPM6 gene
- Isolated recessive hypomagnesemia with normocalciuria
- Mutations in the epidermal growth factor (EGF) gene
- Mutations in the FXYD2 gene encoding γ-subunit of Na/K-ATPase
- Hypercalcemia. Increased Mg^{2+} excretion
- Isolated dominant hypomagnesemia with hypocalciuria
- Diabetic ketoacidosis. Increased Mg^{2+} excretion
- Volume expansion leading to increased GFR with increased Na^+, water, and Mg^{2+} excretion
- Hyperaldosteronism. Causes enhanced Mg^{2+} excretion.

Medicines

Diuretics:

- Including osmotic, loop, and thiazide diuretics, cause renal Mg2+ wasting and inhibition of TRPM6 by thiazides.

Antibiotics:

- Aminoglycosides cause activation of CaSR receptors and renal Mg2+ wasting
- Amphotericin-B causes renal Mg2+ wasting (unknown molecular mechanism)
- Pentamidine reduces Mg2+ reabsorption probably in distal convoluted tubules of nephrons
- Foscarnet makes complexes with Mg2+ and Ca2+.

Antineoplastics:

- Cisplatin renal Mg2+ wasting
- EGF receptor antagonist (Cetuximab) inhibits the activity of TRPM6
- Proton pump inhibitors. Potential pathways include (1) reduced intestinal absorption due to achlorhydria, (2) enhanced intestinal secretion and loss in stool, (3) lowered intestinal TRPM6 activity due to inhibition of H/K-ATPase, and (4) decreased transport by paracellular transport pathway
- Cyclosporine and tacrolimus. Inhibit TRPM6 activity
- Rapamycin causes renal Mg2+ wasting due to inhibition of Na/K/2Cl and TRPM6 activity.

Miscellaneous:

- Hyperthyroidism causes cellular shift
- "Hungry bone syndrome" signifies uptake by bones following parathyroidectomy
- Neonatal hypomagnesemia due to renal loss in diabetic pregnant mothers, use of stool softeners by pregnant mothers, malabsorption/or hyperparathyroidism in mothers.

Remember "**Low Mag**"
• Limited intake Mg+ (starvation)
• Other electrolyte issues cause low mag levels (**hypOkalemia**, **hypOcalcemia**)
• Wasting Magnesium from kidneys (loop- and thiazide diuretics & cyclosporine. Stimulate the kidneys to waste Mg)
• Malabsorption issues (Crohn's, Celiac, proton-pump inhibitors drugs "Prilosec, Nexium, Protonix" ...drug family ending in "prazole" Omeprazole, diarrhea/vomiting)
• Alcohol (due to poor dietary intake, alcohol stimulates the kidneys to excrete Mg, acute pancreatitis)
• Glycemic issues (Diabetic Ketoacidosis, insulin administration)

Clinical Manifestations

Clinical symptoms of hypomagnesemia are also impossible to discern from hypocalcemia. This challenge is due to hypomagnesemia, hypocalcemia, and hypokalemia.

Manifestations are mainly related to neuromuscular and cardiovascular processes.

- Chvostek's sign
- Nausea
- Trousseau's sign
- Vomiting
- Tremors
- Apathy
- Muscle fasciculations
- Weakness
- Hyperreflexia
- Anorexia
- Seizures
- Mental retardation
- Depression
- Psychosis
- Prolonged QT interval
- Cardiac arrhythmias
- Decreased myocardial contractility
- Hypertension
- Sudden death

146

Remember **"Twitching"**
Trousseau's sign (positive due to hypocalcemia)
Weak respirations
Irritability
"Torsades de pointes" (abnormal heart rhythm that leads to sudden cardiac death. seen in alcoholism) **T**etany (seizures)
Cardiac changes (moderate loss: Tall T-waves and depressed ST segments*** severe loss: prolonged PR & QT interval (prolong of QT interval increases patient's risk for Torsades-de-pointes) with widening QRS complex, flattened t-waves, **C**hvostek's sign (positive, which goes along with hypocalcemia)
Hypertension, **H**yperreflexia
Involuntary movements
Nausea
GI issues (decreased bowel sounds and mobility)

Diagnosis
Step 1

• History: GI and renal deficiency of Mg 2+ are the two most common disorders of hypomagnesemia. As a consequence, think of diarrhea or malabsorption or medications that induce renal Mg2+ deficiency.

• In children, family history is critical.

Step 2

• Physical examination is essential. Elicit signs and symptoms of hypomagnesemia.

Step 3

• Order specific tests, including Ca2+, phosphate, and albumin.
• If the cause is not evident, obtain 24 h of Mg2+ urine and creatinine. If it is not possible to extract 24 hours of urine, measure FEMg in spot urine.
• If FEMg is <5 percent, assume GI or cellular uptake losses.
• If FEMg is >5 percent, assume renal failure.

• Serum [Mg2+] can be normal, considering the overall body deficiency of Mg2+. In such cases, some doctors prescribe an Mg2+-loading test (2.4 mg/kg of elemental Mg2+ in D5W to be injected over 4 hours, and <70% of urinary excretion suggests Mg2+ deficiency) to measure the overall body deficit. This test is not consistently recommended due to high false-positives (diarrhea, malabsorption) and false-negatives (renal Mg2+ wasting).
The following algorithm may help to evaluate hypomagnesemia:

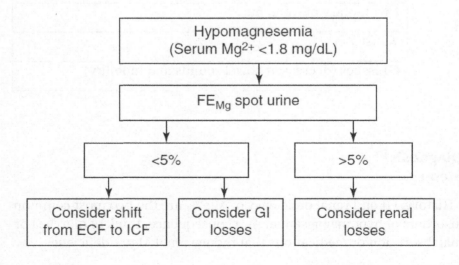

Treatment

Hypomagnesemia management relies on the severity of the symptoms. Symptoms typically arise when the serum [Mg2+] is <1.0 mg/dL. Hypocalcemia and hypokalemia coexist with hypomagnesemia. It is also difficult to distinguish different clinical forms of hypomagnesemia. It is thus advisable to treat hypomagnesemia first and then other electrolyte disorders. In some individuals, both calcium gluconate and KCl are required to replenish both electrolyte deficits after Mg2+ administration. Various magnesium salts are used for oral treatment, and only magnesium sulfate is used parenterally.

Acute Treatment

Severe Symptomatic Hypomagnesemia

• Intravenous magnesium sulfate (2 mL diluted in 100 mL of regular saline) for 10 min. in patients with arrhythmias, seizures, or extreme neuromuscular irritability, and hemodynamically unstable patients.

• Continue IV therapy with 2 mL of magnesium sulfate per 3–4 h until the serum [Mg2+] is greater than 1.0 mg/dL.
• Note that much of the magnesium administered is excreted in patients with normal renal function. Serum creatinine levels should also be followed to prevent hypermagnesemia.

• A dose reduction (50%) is required in patients with compromised renal function.

Hemodynamically Stable Patients with Symptomatic Hypomagnesemia (≥ 1.0 mg/dL)

• Intravenous(IV) magnesium sulfate (4–8 mL dissolved in 1 L of regular saline or D5W) in a total of 12–24 h. This dosage can be repeated if required until the serum [Mg2+] is greater than 1.0 mg/dL.

Special Groups of Patients Requiring Intravenous Magnesium Sulfate

• Patients requiring complete parenteral nutrition, post-op patients, and patients with diarrheal disorders need IV magnesium to ensure near-normal serum [Mg^{2+}]. Often, patients with serious renal failure need IV treatment.

Chronic Treatment

• Foster magnesium-rich foods such as green leafy vegetables, beef, fish, nuts, etc.
• Oral treatment is recommended if the medicine is necessary.
• There are many oral formulations available, many of which have adverse effects, such as diarrhea and abdominal cramping or discomfort.

• The option of oral preparation depends on both the practitioner and the patients.
• The dosage and duration depend on the tolerability of the patients.
• The usual dosage is 240–1,000 mg of elemental Mg^{2+} in split doses a day, in patients with proper renal function.

• Sustained-release preparations (magnesium chloride, Mag Delay, Slow-Mag or magnesium lactate, Mag-Tab SR) are favored due to slow absorption and limited renal excretion Mg^{2+}.
• Magnesium oxide (400–1,200 mg daily) if there is no slow-release preparation available.
• Amiloride should be used in patients with Mg^{2+} renal waste and normal renal function.
• Use medications that facilitate the excretion of Mg^{2+} with caution.

Encourage foods which are abundant in Magnesium.
A good mnemonic to remember these is:

Always Get Plenty of Foods Containing Large Numbers of Magnesium
• Avocado
• Green vegetables
• Peanut Butter, potatoes, pork
• Oatmeal
• Fish (canned white tuna/mackerel)
• Cauliflower, chocolate (dark)
• Legumes
• Nuts
• Oranges
• Milk

Hypermagnesemia

Hypermagnesemia is defined as serum [Mg2+] >2.7 mg/dL. The kidney can preserve serum [Mg2+] within a reasonable range by increasing its excretion, in circumstances of excess Mg2+ intake. As a result, the drop in glomerular filtration rate (GFR) seen in chronic kidney disease is likely to be the most frequent cause of hypermagnesemia. The other primary cause is the exogenous load of Mg2+. Excess amounts of Mg2+ may occur when a patient with pre-eclampsia (a disorder characterized by proteinuria and hypertension in the last trimester of pregnancy) is administered with magnesium sulfate or when individuals take Mg2+-containing antacids or enemas. Pre-eclampsia/eclampsia babies born to mothers who have been treated with magnesium may experience hypermagnesemia. Older adults are especially vulnerable to Mg2+ toxicity because of reduced kidney activity due to aging and heavy use of Mg2+-containing drugs and vitamins. Individuals with familial hypocalciuric hypercalcemia may have elevated levels of Mg2+. Patients with acromegaly and patients with adrenal insufficiency may have hypermagnesemia.

Remember "**MAG**"
Magnesium-containing antacids and laxatives
Addison's disease (adrenal insufficiency)
Glomerular filtration insufficiency (<30mL/min) in renal failure.

Clinical Manifestations
Systemic diseases

- Acute kidney injury ↓ Excretion
- Chronic kidney disease stages 4–5 ↓ Excretion
- Familial hypocalciuric hypercalcemia ↓ Excretion
- Adrenal insufficiency ↑Renal absorption
- Acromegaly ↓ Excretion

- Administration of Mg2+ to treat hypomagnesemia. Exogenous load and ↓ excretion
- Mg2+-containing laxatives. Exogenous load and ↓ excretion
- Mg2+-containing antacids. Exogenous load and ↓ excretion
- Epsom salts. Exogenous load and ↓ excretion.

Mg2+ load in patients with normal GFR

- Treatment of pre-eclampsia/eclampsia. Exogenous load
- Treatment of hypertension in pregnant women. Exogenous load and↓ excretion
- Infants born to mothers treated with Mg2+ for pre-eclampsia/eclampsia. Transfer from mother to fetus
- Seawater ingestion or drowning. Exogenous load (normal seawater 14 mg/dL; Dead Sea water [the salt lake] 394 mg/dL).

Signs and symptoms of Hypermagnesemia

Two organ systems are greatly affected by hypermagnesemia: the neuromuscular and cardiovascular systems.

Signs/symptoms	Serum [Mg2+] (mg/dL)
Nausea and vomiting	3.6–6.0
Sedation, hyporeflexia, muscle weakness	4.8–8.4
Bradycardia, hypotension	6.0–12.0
Absent reflexes, respiratory paralysis, coma	12.0–18.0
Cardiac arrest	> 18.0

Every system of the body is "**Lethargic.**"
Lethargy (profound)
EKG changes with prolonged PR & QT interval and widened QRS complex
Tendon reflexes absent/grossly diminished

Hypotension
Arrhythmias (bradycardia, heart blocks)
Respiratory arrest
GI issues (nausea, vomiting)
Impaired breathing (due to skeletal weakness)
Cardiac arrest

Treatment
Asymptomatic Patient:

• Removal of the cause will normalize plasma [Mg^{2+}].

• If the plasma concentration does not return to normal, volume expansion and a loop diuretic promote Mg^{2+} excretion in a patient with normal GFR.

Symptomatic Patient:

• Intravenous calcium gluconate (15 mg/kg) should be given over a 4-h period. Ca^{2+} antagonizes the neuromuscular and cardiovascular effects of hypermagnesemia.

• For a patient with renal insufficiency, hemodialysis using an Mg^{2+}-free dialysate is the treatment of choice. Since Mg^{2+} is removed by hemodialysis, this treatment provides an efficient means of lowering plasma [Mg^{2+}] within a short period.

Chapter 8
Serum Chloride

Chloride is the prevalent anion in extracellular space. It retains cell integrity by its effects on osmotic pressure and water equilibrium, and maintains an acid-base balance. The normal chloride needs for adults are 80-120 mEq/d as sodium chloride (NaCl).

Normal values:

Adult/elderly	98-106 mEq/L or 98-106 mmol/L (SI units)
Child	90-110 mEq/L
Newborn	96-106 mEq/L
Premature baby	95-110 mEq/L

Possible critical values: < 80 or > 115 mEq/L

Chloride is an extracellular fluid anion that plays an important role in maintaining the normal acid-base equilibrium and retaining water balance and serum osmolality and sodium. It occurs primarily as sodium chloride or hydrochloric acid. Hyperchloremia implies a massive level of serum chloride, and hypochloremia means a low level of serum chloride. Chloride typically represents increases in sodium, except in acid-based disorders where changes in chloride are sodium-independent.

Serum chloride helps to assess normal or high-anion gap metabolic acidosis, and make the differentiation between hypercalcemia secondary to primary hyper-parathyroidism, versus hypercalcemia secondary to malignancy (elevated vs. low chloride, respectively). It is typically used along with sodium, potassium, and CO_2 to assess the electrolyte, acid-base, and water balance.

Hypochloremia

Hypochloremic alkalosis develops from either insufficient chloride consumption or excessive chloride waste. Whereas low chloride consumption is very rare, high chloride-loss sometimes occurs in hospital patients, usually due to diuretic therapy or nasogastric tube suctioning. Diarrhea, when watery, is highly suggestive of chloride-losing diarrhea.

Signs and symptoms

Hypochloremia itself has no signs or manifestations at all. Instead, the resulting signs and symptoms arise from electrolyte imbalances or root causes of hypochloremia.

Symptoms that can be observed in fetuses and neonates are the following:

- Prenatal polyhydramnios
- Prolonged neonatal jaundice
- Lack of meconium or delayed meconium
- Hypotonia and lethargy without sepsis
- Abdominal distension of unknown etiology.

Symptoms that can be observed in infants are the following:

- Repeated vomiting
- Failure to thrive
- Constipation
- Watery diarrhea
- Polyuria
- Salty taste upon being kissed
- Central nervous system (CNS) dysfunctions (e.g. lethargy, confusion, or seizure)
- Neuromuscular symptoms (e.g. weakness and muscle cramps)
- Other symptoms (e.g. abdominal distention, dry skin, apathy, loss of interest, and frequent hospital admissions for recurrent dehydration).

General physical findings may include the following:

- Small size for age
- Signs of chronic dehydration (e.g. skin-tenting as well as poor peripheral perfusion).

The clinical manifestations of the CNS can include the following:

- Confusion
- Disorientation
- Apathy
- Seizure
- Excessive sleeping
- Stupor.

Abdominal symptoms can include:

- Scaphoid or distended belly (depending on the cause of the hypochloremic alkalosis)
- Peristaltic waves in children with chloride-loss diarrhea (CLD)
- Intensified bowel sounds in patients with CLD
- Hard stool in patients with Bartter Syndrome
- Hepatomegaly: (suggesting cystic fibrosis)
- Musculoskeletal findings include muscle loss, atrophy, and hypotonia.
- Respiratory findings include shallow respiration and hypopnea in seriously affected infants.

Diagnosis

Laboratory findings that may be beneficial include the following:

- Amniocentesis
- Serum electrolyte levels; blood pH; serum bicarbonate, uric acid, hemoglobin, renin, and aldosterone
- Urine and stool studies; urinary chloride, sodium, and potassium concentrations; urinary calcium-creatinine and uric acid-creatinine ratios; stool electrolytes (when measurable)
- Tests for kidney and liver functions
- Genetic Analysis
- Ultrasonography.

Ultrasonography can be of use for the following reasons:

- Prenatal - Detection of small prenatal polyhydramnios and measurement of intestinal fluid content
- Postnatal - Assessment of fluid-filled intestines, renal echogenicity, nephrocalcinosis, medullar or diffuse calcinosis, and renal development and growth

- A physiologic study of renal tubules by performing maximal free water clearance during hypotonic saline diuresis is indicated.

Additional findings that can be considered would include the following:

- Wrist radiography
- Upper gastrointestinal (GI) series
- Computed tomography (CT) of the brain
- Magnetic resonance imaging (MRI) of the brain
- Electroencephalography (EEG)
- Renal nuclear scanning
- Renal biopsy.

Management

Substitution of electrolytes with chloride salts is the most effective method of therapy. Nonsteroidal anti-inflammatory drugs (NSAIDs) have been used in people with Bartter's syndrome. Hydrochloric acid and carbonic anhydrase inhibitors can be used in some acute cases.

Initial medical therapy (≤ 6 hours) includes the following:

- Dehydration status and extent of hypochloremia, hypokalemia, hyponatremia, and metabolic alkalosis
- In the event of trauma, aggressive resuscitation of isotonic fluid, ideally natural saline
- Drawing of blood and urine samples for electrolyte testing
- Maintenance therapy (7-72 hours) relies on how much progress happened following initial treatment. The goal is to increase serum potassium concentration very slowly as the amount of serum bicarbonate drops.

Long-term management (>72 hours) should contain the following:

- Discontinuation of intravenous (IV) fluids
- Oral administration (q6-8h) of the measured daily quantities of chloride, sodium, and potassium required to correct serum electrolyte levels.
- Other treatment procedures, as applicable, for the disorder determined to be the primary cause of hypochloremic alkalosis

- Surgical or endoscopic operation is not mandatory except under limited circumstances (e.g. when the cause of hypochloremic alkalosis is an upper GI tract abnormality).

Dietary measures that may be considered include the following:

- Kilojoule intake appropriate for the patient's catabolic status
- Additional protein, to prevent malnutrition
- Additional fat, depending on the individual patient's requirements
- Multivitamins and hematinic agents, as required
- Supplemental trace elements (e.g. zinc), as necessary
- High-sodium and high-potassium diets for patients with Bartter syndrome or CLD.

LOW! "ADD a PINK CARMA SCAR"
A=ADDISON'S DISEASE
D=DIARRHOEA
D=DIURETICS
P=PARACENTESIS
I=IRRITABILITY
N=SODIUM LOW
K=POTASSIUM LOW
C=CYSTIC FIBROSIS
A=ACIDOSIS
R=RESPIRATORY
M=METABOLIC
A=ALKALOSIS
S=SEIZURES
C=COMA
A=ARRYTHMIAS
R=RESPIRATORY ARREST

Hyperchloremia

Hyperchloremia is an electrolyte imbalance in which the amount of chloride ions in the blood is raised. The standard chloride serum range is 96 to 106 mEq/L. Consequently, chloride levels at or below 110 mEq/L typically suggest renal failure, as blood is a chloride regulator.

Signs and symptoms:

There are no specific symptoms of hyperchloremia. However, several irregularities can be noted or functions impaired, involving loss of electrolyte-free fluid, depletion of hypotonic fluid, or increased sodium chloride administration. These disorders are caused by diarrhea, dehydration, elevated sodium chloride consumption, renal impairment, diuretic use, and diabetes.

- Dehydration - due to diarrhea, vomiting, sweating
- Cardiovascular dysfunction - as a result of increased sodium chloride intake
- Hypertension - because of increased sodium chloride intake
- Edema - owing to an influx of sodium into the body
- Weakness - caused by loss of fluids
- Thirst - as a result of the loss of fluids
- Kussmaul breathing - owing to high ion concentrations, loss of fluids, or kidney failure
- High blood sugar - caused by diabetes
- Hyperchloremic metabolic acidosis - because of severe diarrhea and/or kidney failure
- Respiratory alkalosis - because of renal dysfunction.

Hyperchloremic metabolic acidosis

Hyperchloremia should not be associated with hyperchloric metabolic acidosis as two main modifications characterize hyperchloric metabolic acidosis:

- Decreased blood pH and bicarbonate levels.
- Increased serum chloride levels.

Instead, individuals with hyperchloric metabolic acidosis are not typically predisposed to hyperchloremia.

A low concentration of plasma bicarbonate (HCO3-) is known as metabolic acidosis, which may be primary or secondary to respiratory alkalosis. Loss of bicarbonate reserves by diarrhea or renal tubular loss contributes to a metabolic acidosis state marked by increased plasma chloride concentrations, and reduced plasma bicarbonate concentrations. Primary metabolic acids that arise due to a pronounced rise in the production of endogenous acids (e.g. lactic or ketoacids) or gradual aggregation of endogenous acids as the excretion is compromised by renal insufficiency, are distinguished by decreased plasma bicarbonate concentrations and increased anion gaps without hyperchloremia.

The initial distinction of metabolic acidosis should include the discovery of the anion difference (AG). This is typically classified as AG = (Na+)-[(HCO3-+Cl-)], in which Na+ is a plasma sodium concentration, HCO3- a bicarbonate concentration, and Cl- a chloride concentration; all quantities in this formula are in mmol/L (mM or mEq/L). The AG meaning is the difference between unmediated cations and anions, i.e., the presence of anions in the plasma that are not measured regularly.

Increased AG is associated with kidney dysfunction, ketoacidosis, lactic acidosis, and toxin ingestion. Typically, it can be detected easily by analyzing the effects of routine plasma chemistry and the clinical image.

Normal AG acidosis is characterized by a lowered bicarbonate concentration, which is compensated by an equal rise in plasma chloride concentration. For this function, it is also known as hyperchloric metabolic acidosis.

This result indicates that Cl-plasma has effectively replaced HCO3-plasma; hyperchloric metabolic acidosis occurs from one of the following conditions:

- Loss of bicarbonate from body fluids by the GI tract or kidneys, with resulting accumulation of chloride
- Defective renal acidification, inability to excrete normal concentrations of metabolically-formed acid (whereby the conjugate base is excreted, as the sodium salt and sodium chloride is retained)
- Adding hydrochloric acid to body fluids
- Adding or producing another acid, with fast titration of bicarbonate and rapid renal excretion of the resulting anion, and substitution of chloride

- Rapid dilution of plasma bicarbonate with saline.

Associated disorders in hyperchloremic acidosis

- Conditions associated with hyperchloremic acidosis include the following:
- Associated gastrointestinal (GI) or renal or autoimmune disorders
- Hereditary disease
- Effects of agents used for treatment (e.g. cardiac complications).

Signs and symptoms of hyperchloremic acidosis

- If acidosis is marked and/or acute, the patient can experience headaches, loss of energy, nausea, and vomiting.
- Increases in minute ventilation of up to 4-to-8-fold can occur in individuals with respiratory compensation.
- Impact on the cardiovascular system includes direct impairment of myocardial contraction (especially at pH < 7.2), tachycardia, and elevated risk of ventricular fibrillation or heart failure, with pulmonary edema. Patients may experience dyspnea on exercise or, in serious cases, on rest.
- Chronic acidemia, as seen in RTA, can lead to a wide variety of skeletal problems. Clinical consequences include osteomalacia (leading to impaired growth), osteitis fibrosa (from secondary hyper-parathyroidism), rickets (in children), and osteomalacia or osteopenia (in adults).
- Significant complications of recurrent RTA (mainly distal, type I) are nephrocalcinosis and urolithiasis.

Workup in hyperchloremic acidosis

- If the cause of the patient's acidosis is not clear from the history and physical evaluation results, the next step is to determine if hyperchloric acidosis is present. The assessments should contain the following:
- Urinary ammonium excretion (urine AG; urine net charge) is inferred from urine AG, also known as urine net charge, where direct ammonium calculation is not feasible.
- Urinary pH - this tends to increase in the presence of large amounts of ammonia in the urine.

- Acid-loading tests - the most common acid-loading test uses ammonium chloride (NH_4Cl)
- Urinary PCO 2 test - the urinary PCO 2 test during alkaline diuresis reflects the rate of proton secretion in the distal tubule.
- Sodium sulfate test: in healthy individuals, the administration of sodium salt of a non-absorbable anion in the presence of sodium-avid states results in negative intratubular potential, and therefore increased secretion of proton and potassium; in patients with either secretive or voltage defect, the urine will not become maximally acidic.
- Furosemide test - the evidence suggests that furosemide promotes distal acidification by boosting distal sodium intake; the results should be interpreted in the same way as the sodium sulfate test.

Management of hyperchloric acidosis

Proximal RTA

Multi-therapy with large amounts of alkali, vitamin D, and potassium supplementation is needed in proximal RTA (PRTA) cases. The normal bicarbonate administration level is 5-15 mEq/kg/d; large amounts of potassium must accompany administration.

Hypokalemic distal RTA

In hypokalemic distal RTA (dRTA), long-term administration of alkali is sufficient to counterbalance the production of endogenous acids and any bicarbonaturia present. Potassium supplements are noted in the presence of hypokalemia.

Hyperkalemic dRTA

In the case of hyperkalemic dRTA, intervention-prone entities such as obstructive uropathy must be identified. In general, distal sodium delivery is enhanced if patients increase their dietary salt ingestion, given that many of these patients have concomitant cardiorenal compromises.

Fluid overload can be overcome by adding furosemide to a high-salt diet. This combined effect encourages distal sodium delivery by making the collection tube impermeable to chloride and increasing sodium exchange for hydrogen and potassium.

HIGH! "MAD as A KIND CUSHING CLOCK"
M=METABOLIC
A=ACIDOSIS
D=DEHYDRATION
AS=ASPIRIN TOXICITY
AK=KUSSMAUL BREATHING
I=INCREASED
N=SODIUM
D=DIABETIC INSIPIDIOUS
CUSHING=CUSHING'S DISEASE
L=LACTATE RINGER
O=ORIENTATION
C=CORTISOL/STEROID
K=KAYEXALATE

Chapter 9
Arterial Blood Gas Analysis (ABGs)

Maintaining normal blood pH requires a variety of organ systems and is dependent on circulatory integrity. It is not unusual, then, that disruption of the acid-base equilibrium will complicate the treatment of a wide variety of diseases and cause damage to many areas of the body. The body has a tremendous capacity to maintain blood pH, but diseases affecting it typically include serious chronic disease or acute critical illness.

Arterial blood gas analysis is the most common procedure conducted by nurses on seriously ill patients in the emergency department, the treatment room, and the intensive care unit. One of the procedure's key aims is determining acid-base status, which is frequently interrupted during serious illness. The body's challenge is that normal metabolism is correlated with the constant development of hydrogen ions (H+) and carbon dioxide (CO_2), all of which help to decrease pH. The process that overcomes this problem and serves to retain normal blood pH (i.e., retaining acid-based homeostasis) is a dynamic synergy of action involving chemical buffers in red cells (erythrocytes), as they circulate.

Normal cell metabolism depends on maintaining blood pH within very narrow limits (7.35-7.45).

Even comparatively minor excursions beyond this standard pH range can have deleterious effects, including the decreased supply of oxygen to tissues, electrolyte disruptions, and changes in heart muscle contractility; survival is unlikely if blood pH is below 6.8 or above 7.8.
To understand how these five components relate to the overall conservation of blood pH, a brief overview of some basic principles will help.

What is an acid?

An acid is an agent that activates hydrogen ions (H+) on dissociation in solution. For instance, hydrochloric acid (HCl) dissociates into hydrogen ions and chloride ions.

$$HCl \longrightarrow H^+ + Cl^-$$

Carbonic acid (H2CO3) disintegrates into hydrogen ions and bicarbonate ions.

$$H_2CO_3 \longrightarrow H^+ + HCO_3^-$$

We differentiate between stronger acids such as hydrochloric acid and weak acids such as carbonic acid. The distinction is that strong acids are more dissociated than weak acids. As a result, the abundance of hydrogen ions in a strong acid is significantly greater than that of a weak acid.

What is the base?

The base is a substance that accepts hydrogen ions in the solution.

For example, the base bicarbonate (HCO3−) uses hydrogen ions to form carbonic acid:

$$HCO_3^- + H^+ \longrightarrow H_2CO_3$$

What is pH?

pH is an evaluation of acidity and alkalinity on a scale of 0-14. Simple water has a pH value of 7 and is neutral (neither acidic nor alkaline). Any solution with a pH 7 or above is termed as alkaline, and below 7 is acidic. Thus, the pH of the blood (7.35-7.45) is slightly alkaline, but the term alkalosis in clinical practice is, somewhat confusingly, used for blood pH greater than 7.45, and the word acidosis is reserved for blood pH less than 7.35.

pH is a gauge of the hydrogen ion concentration (H+). The two are related corresponding to the following equation:

$pH = -\log_{10}[H^+]$
where [H+] is the number of hydrogen ions in moles per liter (mol/L)
From this equation
pH 7.4 = H+ ion concentration of 40 nmol/L pH 7.0 = H+ ion strength of 100 nmol/L AND pH 6.0 = H+ ion concentration of 1000 nmol/L

It is evident that:

- The two parameters change inversely; as the concentration of hydrogen ions increases, the pH decreases.
- Due to the logarithmic relationship, a major change in hydrogen ion concentration is a minor pH change. For example, doubling the concentration of hydrogen ions causes the pH to fall by just 0.3.

What is a buffer? – the bicarbonate buffer system

Buffers are chemicals that limit the pH alteration that happens as acids are introduced, by 'mopping up' hydrogen ions. A buffer is a weak acid solution with a conjugate base. The blood's primary buffer system is a weak acid, carbonic acid (H_2CO_3), and its conjugate base is bicarbonate (HCO_3-). To illustrate how this method minimizes pH changes, assume we apply a strong acid, e.g. HCl, to the bicarbonate buffer:

The acid dissociates and releases hydrogen ions:

$HCl \longrightarrow H^+ + Cl^-$

The bicarbonate buffer then 'absorbs' hydrogen ions, producing carbonic acid:

$HCO_3^- + H^+ \longrightarrow H_2CO_3$ (carbonic acid)

The key argument is that since the hydrogen ions from HCl have been introduced into the mild carbonic acid that does not dissolve as quickly, the overall amount of hydrogen ions in the solution, and the pH, do not change greatly in the presence of the buffer.

Although the buffer substantially minimizes pH shift, it does not remove pH change, and even the weak acid (like carbonic acid) disassociates to some degree. The buffer solution's pH depends on the relative strengths of the weak acid and its conjugate base.

The equation is as following:

pH = $6.1 + \log ([HCO_3^-] / [H_2CO_3])$

Where $[HCO_3^-]$ represents the concentration of bicarbonate, while $[H_2CO_3]$ is the concentration of carbonic acid.

This relation, known as the Henderson-Hasselbalch equation, shows that pH is calculated by the ratio of base (HCO_3-) content to acid (H_2CO_3) content.

As hydrogen ions add up to the bicarbonate buffer:

$$H^+ + HCO_3^- \longrightarrow H_2CO_3$$

Bicarbonate (base) is used (concentration decreases), and carbonic acid is formed (concentration increases). If hydrogen ions continued to be added, all bicarbonate would gradually be consumed (converted to carbonic acid), and there would eventually be no buffering impact – pH would then decrease significantly if more acid were added.

However, if carbonic acid could be continually eliminated from the environment and bicarbonate constantly regenerated, the buffering power and the pH could be retained despite the continuing addition of hydrogen ions.

In essence, the lungs ensure the removal of carbonic acid (as carbon dioxide), and the kidneys ensure continuous regeneration of bicarbonate.

The lungs' role depends on the bicarbonate buffering system's singular characteristic, which is carbonic acid's ability to be converted to carbon dioxide as well as water.

The following equation describes the relationship between all the bicarbonate-buffering mechanism components as it functions within the body.

$$H^+ + HCO_3^- \longleftrightarrow H_2CO_3 \longleftrightarrow H_2O + CO_2$$

It is important to remember that the reactions are reversible. The path depends on the relative concentration of each factor. For instance, an increase in the concentration of carbon dioxide forces interacts to the left with an increase in the carbonic acid formation and, eventually, hydrogen ions.

This highlights the acid potential of carbon dioxide and leads to the essential contribution that lungs and red cells make to the overall acid-base balance.

Lung role, CO_2 transport, and acid-base balance

The known concentrations of CO_2 in the blood, which is necessary for normal acid-base equilibrium, represents the balance between that created by tissue and cell metabolism and that excreted by the lungs in the exhaled air.

By altering the rate at which carbon dioxide is released into the atmosphere, the lungs maintain the blood's carbon dioxide content. Carbon dioxide is diffused from tissue cells to the capillary fluid. A limited amount dissolves in blood plasma, and the rest is transported, unchanged, to the lungs.

However, most diffuses into red cells, where it combines with water to form carbonic acid. The acid dissociates, with the production of hydrogen ions and bicarbonate. Hydrogen ions interact with deoxygenated hemoglobin (hemoglobin serves as a barrier here), avoid a harmful decrease in cell pH, and bicarbonate moves over a concentration gradient from the red cell to the plasma.

Consequently, a major part of the carbon dioxide produced in the tissues is transported to the lungs as bicarbonate in the blood plasma.

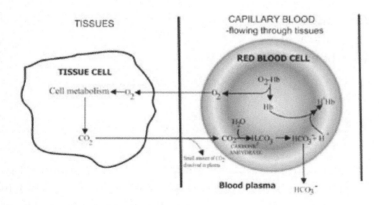

CO_2 is formed in tissues, and is converted to bicarbonate for transport to the lungs.

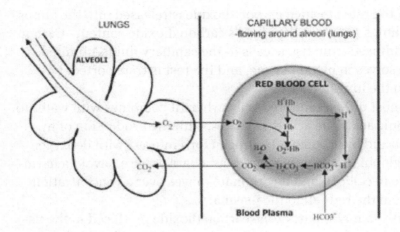

- H⁺ = hydrogen ions
- Hb = hemoglobin
- O_2-Hb = oxyhemoglobin
- H⁺Hb = reduced hemoglobin, which acts as a buffer
- CO_2 = carbon dioxide
- H_2CO_3 = carbonic acid
- HCO_3^- = bicarbonate ions
- O_2 = oxygen

At the lungs, bicarbonate is converted back to CO_2 and eliminated by the lungs. The mechanism is reversed at the alveoli of the lungs. Hydrogen ions are displaced from hemoglobin by taking oxygen from the inspired air. Hydrogen ions are now buffered with bicarbonate, released from plasma back to the red cell, and carbonic acid is formed. If the concentration of this increases, it is converted into water and carbon dioxide. Finally, carbon dioxide disperses through the concentration gradient from red cells to alveoli, for excretion in the expired air.

Respiratory chemoreceptors located in the brain stem respond to variations in the concentration of carbon dioxide in the blood, triggering increased ventilation (breathing) as carbon dioxide concentration increases, and reduced ventilation when carbon dioxide decreases.

Kidneys and acid-base balance

Normal cellular metabolism results in the continuous production of hydrogen ions. We have seen that the bicarbonate buffer in blood minimizes their effect by combining with these hydrogen ions; however, buffering is only effective in the short term because, eventually, hydrogen ions must be eliminated from the body. Furthermore, the bicarbonate that is used to buffer hydrogen ions must be continuously replaced. These two functions, the removal of hydrogen ions and bicarbonate regeneration, are performed by the kidneys. Renal tubular cells are rich in the enzyme carbonic anhydrase, promoting carbonic acid production from carbon dioxide and water. Carbonic acid dissociates with bicarbonate and hydrogen ions. The bicarbonate is reabsorbed into the blood, and the hydrogen ions pass into the lumen of the tubule and are expelled from the body in the urine. This urinary elimination relies on buffers' availability, especially phosphate and ammonia ions in the urine.

Disturbances of Acid-Base Balance

Most of the acid-base disruptions are caused by:

- Disease or injury to organs (kidney, lung, brain), the normal function of which is essential for acid-based homeostasis.
- A condition that induces abnormally-increased development of metabolic acids, so that homeostatic processes are overloaded.
- Medicinal intervention (e.g. mechanical ventilation, some drugs).

Arterial blood gases are blood samples used to diagnose and track acid-based disruptions. Three parameters calculated during the blood gas study, arterial blood pH (pH), partial carbon dioxide pressure in arterial blood ($pCO_2(a)$), and bicarbonate concentration (HCO3−), are of critical importance (see Table I for comparison [normal range]). The results of these three make the classification of acid-base disruptions into one of four etiological categories:

- Respiratory acidosis
- Respiratory alkalosis
- Metabolic acidosis
- Metabolic alkalosis.

	Adults	Neonates
pH	7.35-7.45	7.30-7.40
pCO_2 (kPa)	4.7-6.0	3.5-5.4
Bicarbonate (mmol/L)	22-28	15-25

Approximate reference (normal) ranges.

To understand how pH, pCO_2(a), and bicarbonate effects are used to describe acid-base disturbances in this way, reference must be made to the Henderson-Hasselbalch equation.

$$pH = 6.1 + \log ([HCO_3^-] / [H_2CO_3])$$

This equation calculates pH and bicarbonate but not carbonic acid; (H2CO3). There is, however, a relationship between pCO_2(a) and H2CO3, which results in the readjustment of the Henderson-Hasselbalch equation for the three parameters (pH, pCO_2(a) and bicarbonate) measured during the blood gas analysis:

$$pH = 6.1 + \log ([HCO_3^-] / (pCO_2(a) \times 0.23))$$

By extracting all constants from this equation, the relationship between the three calculated parameters can be described more simply:

pH $\propto$ [HCO$_3^-$] / pCO_2(a)

This relationship, crucial for understanding all that follows acid-base disturbances, states that arterial blood pH is proportional to bicarbonate concentration ratio to pCO_2(a). It allows the following deductions:

- pH remains normal as long as the ratio [HCO3−]: pCO_2(a) remains normal.
- pH increases (i.e., alkalosis occurs) as either [HCO3−] increases or pCO_2(a) decreases.
- PH reduces (i.e., acidosis occurs) as either [HCO3−] decreases or pCO_2(a) increases.
- If *relatively the same amount increases both pCO₂(a) and [HCO3−]*, the ratio, and therefore the pH, is normal.
- If the same amount decreases both pCO_2(a) and [HCO3−], the ratio and the pH are normal.

172

- Acid-based disturbances mainly affect either $pCO_2(a)$, in which case they are referred to as respiratory disorders or [HCO3−], in which case they are referred to as non-respiratory or metabolic disorders:
- If the main disruption is elevated $pCO_2(a)$ (which causes acidosis − see above), the disorder is called respiratory acidosis.
- If the main disturbance is decreased $pCO_2(a)$ (which induces alkalosis, see above), the disease is called respiratory alkalosis.
- If the main disorder is associated with decreased bicarbonate (which occurs in acidosis, see above), it is termed metabolic acidosis.
- If the main change is associated with elevated bicarbonate (which results in alkalosis − see above), the disorder is termed metabolic alkalosis.

Chapter 10
Causes of Acid-Base Disturbances

Respiratory acidosis – (High pCO_2(a), low pH)

Respiratory acidosis is characterized by a rise in pCO_2(a) due to poor alveolar ventilation (hypoventilation) and, subsequently, a decrease in the removal of CO_2 from the blood. Respiratory disorders, such as bronchopneumonia, emphysema, asthma, and persistent obstructive airway disease, can be associated with ventilation low enough to induce respiratory acidosis.

Any medications (e.g. morphine and barbiturates) can induce respiratory acidosis by depressing the brain's respiratory center. Injury, or trauma, to the chest wall and muscles involved in breathing mechanics, can reduce ventilation rate. This describes respiratory acidosis, which can exacerbate polio, Guillain-Barre syndrome, and the healing of serious injuries to the lung.

Respiratory alkalosis – (low pCO_2(a), High pH)

On the other hand, respiratory alkalosis is characterized by reduced pCO_2(a) due to excessive alveolar ventilation and excessive removal of CO_2 from the blood. Reduced oxygen in the blood (hypoxemia) stimulates the respiratory center, resulting in respiratory alkalosis. Examples include extreme anemia, pulmonary embolism, and adult respiratory syndrome. Hyperventilation necessary to induce pulmonary alkalosis can be a symptom of anxiety attacks and a reaction to extreme pain. One of the less pleasant characteristics of salicylate (aspirin) is its stimulating effect on the respiratory center. This result is due to respiratory alkalosis that happens after an overdose of salicylate. In the end, over-enthusiast mechanical ventilation will cause respiratory alkalosis.

Metabolic acidosis – (low HCO$_3^-$, low pH)

Reduced bicarbonate is often a part of metabolic acidosis. This occurs for one of two reasons: increased bicarbonate use in buffering, abnormal acid loading, or increased bicarbonate loss from the body. Diabetic ketoacidosis and lactic acidosis are two disorders characterized by overproduction of metabolic acids and bicarbonate depletion. In the first example, abnormally elevated blood concentrations of keto acids (b-hydroxybutyric acid and acetoacetic acid) represent serious metabolic abnormalities caused by insulin deficiency.

All cells produce lactic acid when they are deficient in oxygen, resulting in increased production of lactic acid and metabolic acidosis in any state in which the supply of oxygen to the tissues is seriously impaired. Examples include cardiac arrest, and any disorders associated with hypovolemic shock (e.g. massive fluid loss). The liver plays a significant role in eliminating the small amount of lactic acid released during normal cell metabolism, so that raised lactic acidosis may be a symptom of liver failure. Abnormal loss of bicarbonate from the body may occur during severe diarrhea. If not investigated, this can lead to metabolic acidosis. Failure to recycle bicarbonate, and excrete hydrogen ions, describes the metabolic acidosis caused by renal failure.

Anion Gap

- Anion Gap (AG) is a derived factor mainly used to measure metabolic acidosis to determine the presence of undesired anions. Anion Gap = $Na^+ - (Cl^- + HCO3^-)$
- The standard anion difference depends on the concentrations of serum phosphate and serum albumin.
- The elevated anion difference indicates the existence of metabolic acidosis.
- The standard anion gap differs with multiple assays but is usually between 4 and 12 mmol/L (if measured by ion-selective electrode; 8 to 16 if measured by the older technique of flame photometry).
- If AG > 30 mmol/L, metabolic acidosis is inevitably present. The anion gap reference range is as follows:
  - 16 ± 4 mEq/L (if the calculation uses potassium)
  - 12 ± 4 mEq/L (if the calculation does not use potassium)
  - If AG 20-29mmol/L so 1/3, does not have metabolic acidosis
  - K + can be added to Na+, but in reality, it provides no benefit.

Albumin and Phosphate

- The typical anion difference is based on serum phosphate and serum albumin.
- Standard AG = 0.2 x [album] (g/L) + 1.5 x [phosphate] (mmol/L).
- Albumin is the major undetermined anion and adds nearly the maximum value of the anion gap.
- Each 1g/L drop in albumin can minimize the anion gap by 0.25 mm.
- Normally elevated anion-gap acidosis in a patient with hypoalbuminemia will present as regular anion gap acidosis.
- This is especially true with patients in ICU, where lower albumin levels are common.

High Anion Gap Metabolic Acidosis (HAGMA)

HAGMA results from the accumulation of organic acids or impaired H+ excretion.

Causes (LTKR)
• Lactate
• Toxins
• Ketones
• Renal

OR

Causes ("CAT MUDPILES")
• CO, CN
• Alcoholic ketoacidosis and starvation ketoacidosis
• Toluene
• Metformin, Methanol
• Uremia
• DKA
• Pyroglutamic acidosis, paracetamol, phenformin, propylene glycol, paraldehyde
• Iron, Isoniazid
• Lactic acidosis
• Ethylene glycol
• Salicylates

Effects of albumin:
- The anion gap may be underestimated in hypoalbuminemia because if albumin fell by 1g/L, then the anion gap decreases by 0.25 mmol
- The corrected AG, which is AG + (0.25 X (40-albumin) expressed in g/L, can be used to counteract the effects of hypoalbuminemia on AG.

Lab tests to consider include:
- glucose, lactate, creatinine and urea, urinary ketones, serum levels of methanol, ethanol, paracetamol, salicylates, and ethylene glycol.
-

Normal Anion Gap Metabolic Acidosis (NAGMA)
NAGMA results from loss of HCO3- from ECF.

Causes ("CAGE")
• **Chloride excess**
• **Acetazolamide/Addisons**
• **GI causes** – diarrhea/vomiting, fistulae (pancreatic, ureters, biliary, small bowel, ileostomy)
• **Extra** – RTA

OR

Causes ("ABCD")
• **Addison's** (adrenal insufficiency)
• **Bicarbonate loss** (GI or Renal)
• **Chloride excess**
• **Diuretics** (Acetazolamide)

The Urinary Anion Gap

Calculate the urinary anion gap to distinguish between the GI and the renal cause of normal anion-gap acidosis. The most common unmediated anion is ammonia, for the urinary anion void. Healthy individuals typically have a gap of 0 to marginally average (< 10 mEq/L). Urine anion differences of more than 20 mEq/L are used in metabolic acidosis where the kidneys cannot excrete ammonia (such as in renal tubular acidosis). If the urine anion difference is negligible or negative, but the serum AG is positive, the possible cause is gastrointestinal (diarrhea or vomiting).

Urinary anion gap $= (Na^+ + K^+) - Cl^-$

- The remaining significant unmeasured ions are NH4+ and HCO3-
- *renal causes:* increased urinary HCO3- excretion thus *increased* urinary AG
- *GI causes:* increased NH4+ excretion, thus *decreased* urinary AG.

Low Anion Gap

Causes:

- Non-random analytical errors (increased Na+, increased viscosity, iodide ingestion, increased lipids)
- The decrease in unmeasured anions (albumin, dilution)
- The increase in unmeasured cations (multi-myeloma (cationic IgG paraprotein), hypercalcemia, hypermagnesaemia, lithium OD, polymixin B)
- Bromide OD (causes falsely elevated chloride measurements).

Metabolic Acidosis

Normal Anion Gap

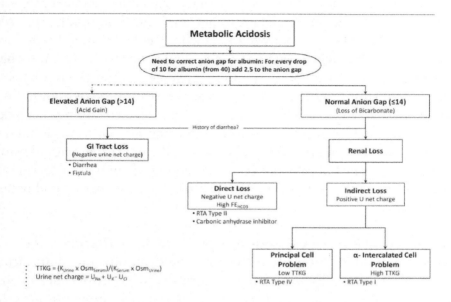

Metabolic Acidosis

Elevated Anion Gap

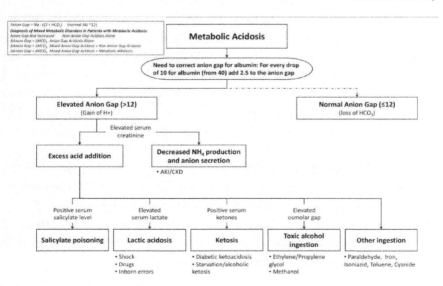

Metabolic Alkalosis – (Increased HCO_3^-, Increased pH)

Bicarbonate is still involved in metabolic alkalosis. Rarely, over-administration of bicarbonate or ingestion of bicarbonate in antacid preparation can induce metabolic alkalosis, but this is normally temporary. Abnormal elimination of hydrogen ions from the body could be the primary concern. Bicarbonate, which would normally be absorbed through the buffering of these missing hydrogen ions, accumulates in the blood. Gastric juice is acidic, and gastric aspiration or another disease phase in which the body loses its gastric material represents a depletion of hydrogen ions. Projectile vomiting of gastric juice, for instance, explains the metabolic alkalosis that can arise in patients with pyloric stenosis. Extreme potassium depletion can induce metabolic alkalosis due to the reciprocal relationship between hydrogen and potassium ions.

Compensation – a consequence of acid-base disturbance

It is important for survival that the pH should not waver too much from normal, and the body will want to restore an unhealthy pH back to normal when the acid-base equilibrium is disrupted. Compensation is the name assigned to this life-saving process. To grasp the compensation, it is necessary to remember that pH is regulated by the ratio [HCO3–]: pCO_2 (a). As long as the ratio is normal, the pH would be normal. Consider a metabolic acidosis patient whose pH is lower because bicarbonate [HCO3–] is low. To compensate for the low [HCO3–] and recover the all-important ratio to normal, the patient should lower his pCO_2 (a). Chemoreceptors in the respiratory area of the brain respond to an increasing concentration of hydrogen ion (low pH), which induces increased breathing (hyperventilation) and thus increased removal of carbon dioxide; pCO_2(a) decreases, and the ratio [HCO3–]: pCO_2(a) returns to zero.

Recompense for metabolic alkalosis in which [HCO3–] is elevated, by comparison, implies respiration depression and thus carbon dioxide retention, such that pCO_2(a) raises to balance the increase in [HCO3–]. However, respiration depression has an unexpected side effect of threatening sufficient tissue oxygenation. Respiratory compensation for metabolic alkalosis is, therefore, minimal.

Primary disturbances of pCO_2(a) (respiratory acidosis and alkalosis) are compensated by renal adjustments of hydrogen ion excretion resulting in changes in [HCO3−] that compensate for the primary change in pCO_2 (a). Renal compensation for respiratory acidosis (raised pCO_2(a)) therefore involves increased bicarbonate reabsorption, and renal compensation for respiratory alkalosis (reduced pCO_2(a)) involves reduced bicarbonate reabsorption.
The following table summarizes the blood gas results that characterize all four acid-base disturbances, before and after compensation.
The "acid-base balance": compensation restores normal pH.

Primary disturbance				
	Respiratory acidosis primary increase in pCO_2	Respiratory alkalosis primary decrease in pCO_2	Metabolic acidosis primary decrease In bicarb.	Metabolic alkalosis primary increase In bicarb.
Some common causes	Emphysema COPD Pneumonia Depression of respiratory center	Hyper-ventilation Anxiety attacks Stimulation of respiratory center in the brain	Renal failure Diabetic ketoacidosis Circulatory failure (lactic acidosis)	Bicarbonate administration Potassium depletion
Compensatory mechanism	RENAL Increase bicarbonate	RENAL decrease bicarbonate	RESPIRATORY decrease pCO_2	RESPIRATORY increase pCO_2 but limited compensation in metabolic alkalosis
Initial blood gas results (uncompensated)	pH decreased pCO_2 increased Bicarbonate normal	pH increased pCO_2 decreased Bicarbonate normal	pH decreased pCO_2 normal Bicarbonate decreased	pH increased pCO_2 normal Bicarbonate increased
Blood gas results after partial compensation	pH decreased but closer to normal pCO_2 increased Bicarbonate increased	pH increased but closer to normal pCO_2 decreased Bicarbonate marginally decreased	pH decreased but closer to normal pCO_2 marginally decreased Bicarbonate decreased	Limited compensation in metabolic alkalosis
Blood gas results after full compensation	pH normal pCO_2 increased Bicarbonate increased	pH normal pCO_2 decreased Bicarbonate decreased	pH normal pCO_2 decreased Bicarbonate decreased	Limited compensation in metabolic alkalosis

Blood gas results in disruptions of acid-base balance

Respiratory compensation for primary metabolic disturbance happens much more quickly than metabolic (renal) compensation for primary respiratory disturbance. In the second example, compensation takes place over days, rather than hours.

If compensation results in the return of pH to normal, then the patient is *fully compensated*. However, in many cases, the compensation returns pH towards normal without actually achieving normality; in such cases, the patient is *partially compensated*.

Metabolic alkalosis is only rarely completely compensated for the factors mentioned above.

Mixed acid-base disturbances

It may be implied from the above discussion that all patients with acid-base disturbance have only one of the four types of acid-base equilibrium, but patients may have more than one disruption, in specific cases. Consider, for example, a patient with chronic lung disease such as emphysema, with long-term partly-compensated respiratory acidosis. If this patient already had diabetes and did not take his usual insulin dosage, and was then in a state of diabetic ketoacidosis, the blood-gas effects would reflect the cumulative effect of both respiratory acidosis and metabolic acidosis.

Such mixed acid-base disruptions are not infrequent, and can be difficult to unrave,l based on arterial blood gas findings alone.

Arterial blood gas analysis results can identify acid-base disturbance and provide valuable information as to its cause.

The acronym **"ROME"** is used as a bits of help to remember the correlation between pH and CO_2.
Respiratory **O**pposite -- In respiratory syndromes, the pH and CO_2 arrows are in opposite directions.
Metabolic **E**qual -- In metabolic syndromes, the PH and CO_2 arrows are in the same direction.

Acid-Base Disturbances and the Body's Reaction

Primary Disturbance	Example	Initial Blood pH	Compensatory Mechanism	Compensatory Change in Blood pH
Metabolic acidosis	Increased synthesis of acid due to diabetic ketoacidosis	Too low	Increased breathing rate to eliminate carbon dioxide	Increases back to normal
Respiratory acidosis	Decreased breathability due to serious chronic lung disease	Too low	Increased urinary acid excretion	Increases back toward normal
Metabolic alkalosis	Loss of stomach acid caused by vomiting	Too high	Decreased breathing rate to retain carbon dioxide	Decreases back toward normal
Respiratory alkalosis	Hyperventilation due to anxiety	Too high	Increased excretion of alkali in the urine	Decreases back toward normal

What is an Arterial Blood Gas (ABG)?

An ABG is a blood test that analyses acidity, or pH, and oxygen (O_2) and carbon dioxide (CO_2) levels in blood from an artery. The procedure is used to assess the patient's lungs' function and how well oxygen can be transported into the blood, and carbon dioxide can be removed. This test is usually conducted in ICU and ER settings; however, ABGs can be done to any patient on any floor, based on their diagnosis.

ABG vs. VBG

A VBG, on the other hand, analyses venous blood and can reliably calculate pH and CO_2, but cannot provide consistent O_2 results. For this cause, arterial monitoring has become the "gold standard" in patients at risk of rapid decompensation, or those with a respiratory element. ABGs are drawn for several reasons. These may include:

- Uncontrolled diabetes
- Ketoacidosis
- Lung Failure
- Kidney Failure
- Shock
- Trauma
- Asthma
- Hemorrhage
- Drug Overdose

- Metabolic Disease
- Chemical Poisoning
- Chronic Obstructive Pulmonary Disease (COPD)
- To confirm if lung-condition treatments are working (patients on ventilators, or oxygen therapy).

How to Draw an ABG

Arterial Blood Gas needs a nurse to take a small blood sample - a complete 1 mL is usually recommended. Blood may be drawn from the wrist, groin, or above the elbow by an arterial stick. The radial artery is the most frequently used for the processing of the sample. However, if necessary, the femoral artery and the brachial artery can be used. If the patient has a pre-existing arterial line, this may be used to provide a sample. Once the blood is obtained, it is either sent to the hospital's central lab for analysis or tested by the respiratory therapist on the unit's blood-gas analyzer. Most ICUs have one on the unit for a quick turnaround. Though arterial samples are best for medical purposes, they raise several problems for nurses and providers. If any individual does not

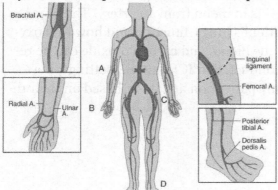

have a good arterial line, the frontline clinician will take the arterial sample. Hospitals allow specially qualified nurses or phlebotomists to practice this skill only after a rigorous training program. If an arterial stick is not accessible to the physician, treatment can be postponed.

Interpretation of ABGs

Interpreting arterial blood gas (ABG) is vital for doctors, nurses, respiratory therapists, and other health-care providers. The understanding of ABG is highly relevant in chronically ill patients. The following six-step method helps to ensure a full understanding of each ABG. You can also notice tables that list frequently observed acid-base disorders. There are several approaches to direct the analysis of the ABG. This topic does not contain some approaches, such as base-excess analysis, or Stewart's strong ion-gap. A description of these approaches can be found in some of the publications suggested. It is uncertain if these alternative approaches give clinically relevant benefits over the "anion gap" strategy.

6-step approach:

Step 1: Evaluate the internal consistency of the obtained values by using the Henderson-Hasselbach equation:

$$[H+] = \frac{24(pCO_2)}{[HCO_3-]} \quad \{pCO_2 \text{ is also shown as } PaCO_2\}$$

If pH and [H+] are contradictory, the blood results of an ABG may not be correct.

pH	Approximate [H+] (nmol/L)
7.00	100
7.05	89
7.10	79
7.15	71
7.20	63
7.25	56
7.30	50

7.35	45
7.40	40
7.45	35
7.50	32
7.55	28
7.60	25
7.65	22

Step 2: Is there an alkalemia, or acidemia?

pH < 7.35 acidemia/acidosis

pH > 7.45 alkalemia/alkalosis

- *Remember: acidosis or alkalosis can be present even though the pH is within the normal range (7.35 – 7.45)*
- *You are going to need to check the pCO_2, HCO3- and anion difference.*

Step 3: Is it respiratory, or metabolic disturbance? What is the relationship between the pH change direction and the pCO_2 change direction? In primary respiratory disorders, pH and pCO_2 change in the opposite direction; in metabolic disorders, pH and pCO_2 change in the same direction.

Acidosis	Respiratory	pH ↓	pCO_2 ↑
Acidosis	Metabolic	pH ↓	pCO_2 ↓
Alkalosis	Respiratory	pH ↑	pCO_2 ↓
Alkalosis	Metabolic	pH ↑	pCO_2 ↑

Step 4: Is there enough compensation for the major disturbance? Usually, the pH does not return to normal (7.35 – 7.45) even after compensation.

Disorder	Expected compensation	Correction factor
Acute respiratory acidosis	Increase in $[HCO_3\text{-}] = \Delta\, pCO_2/10$	± 3
Chronic respiratory acidosis (3-5 days)	Increase in $[HCO_3\text{-}] = 3.5(\Delta\, pCO_2/10)$	
Acute respiratory alkalosis	Reduction in $[HCO_3\text{-}] = 2(\Delta\, pCO_2/10)$	
Chronic respiratory alkalosis	Reduction in $[HCO_3\text{-}] = 5(\Delta\, pCO_2/10)$ to $7(\Delta\, pCO_2/10)$	
Metabolic acidosis	$pCO_2 = (1.5 \times [HCO3\text{-}]) + 8$	± 2
Metabolic alkalosis	Increase in $pCO_2 = 40 + 0.6(\Delta HCO3\text{-})$	-

If the reported compensation is not the predicted compensation, more than one acid-base condition is likely to occur.

Step 5: Assess the anion gap (in case of metabolic acidosis):
AG= [Na+]-([Cl-] + [HCO$_3$-])-12 ± 2

- The standard anion gap is around 12 mEq/L.
- In patients with hypoalbuminemia, the usual anion gap is less than 12 mEq/L; the "normal" anion gap in patients with hypoalbuminemia is around 2.5 mEq/L lower with every 1 gm/dL drop in plasma albumin concentration (for example, a patient with plasma albumin of 2.0 gm/dL will be approximately 7 mEq/L).
- If the anion gap is higher, consider measuring the osmolal gap to be incompatible with clinical conditions.
- When elevation in AG is not clarified in a simple case (DKA, lactic acidosis, renal failure), then ingestion of toxic substances is a concern.
  - OSM gap = measured OSM − (2[Na+] - glucose/18 − BUN/2.8
- The OSM gap should be < 10.

187

Step 6: Where there is an increased anion gap, evaluate the relationship between increasing the anion gap and decreasing [HCO3-].

Evaluate the ratio of the change in the anion gap (ΔAG) to the change in [HCO3-] ($\Delta[HCO_3\text{-}]$): $\Delta AG/\Delta[HCO_3\text{-}]$

This ratio must be between 1.0 and 2.0 if there is an uncomplicated anion gap in metabolic acidosis.

If this ratio falls outside this range, another metabolic disorder is present:

- If $\Delta AG/\Delta[HCO_3\text{-}] < 1.0$, a concurrent non-anion gap, metabolic acidosis is likely to occur.
- If $\Delta AG/\Delta[HCO_3\text{-}] > 2.0$, Concurrent metabolic alkalosis is likely to take place.

It is important to remember the expected "normal" anion gap for your patient by adjusting for hypoalbuminemia (see **Step 5**, above).

Characteristics of acid-base disturbances

Disorder	pH	Primary problem	Compensation
Metabolic acidosis	↓	↓ in HCO_3-	↓ in pCO_2
Metabolic alkalosis	↑	↑ in HCO_3-	↑ in pCO_2
Respiratory acidosis	↓	↑ in pCO_2	↑ in [HCO_3-]
Respiratory alkalosis	↑	↓ in pCO_2	↓ in [HCO_3-]

Selected etiologies of respiratory acidosis

• Airway obstruction - Upper - Lower
• COPD
• asthma
• other obstructive lung diseases
• CNS depression
• Sleep-disordered breathing (OSA or OHS)
• Neuromuscular impairment

• Ventilatory restriction
• Increased CO_2 production: shivering, rigors, seizures, malignant hyperthermia, hypermetabolism, increased intake of carbohydrates
• Incorrect mechanical ventilation settings.

Selected etiologies for respiratory alkalosis
• CNS stimulation: fever, fear, pain, anxiety, CVA, cerebral edema, brain trauma, brain tumor, CNS infection
• Hypoxemia or hypoxia: lung disease, profound anemia, low FiO2
• Stimulation of chest receptors: pulmonary edema, pleural effusion, pneumonia, pneumothorax, pulmonary embolus
• Drugs, hormones: salicylates, catecholamines, progestins medroxyprogesterone,
• Pregnancy, sepsis, hyperthyroidism, liver disease
• Incorrect mechanical ventilation.

Selected causes of metabolic alkalosis

• Hypovolemia with Cl- reduction	
• GI loss of H+	
	▪ Vomiting, villous adenoma, gastric suction, diarrhea with chloride-rich fluid
• Renal loss H+	
	▪ Loop and thiazide diuretics, post-hypercapnia (particularly after the institution of mechanical ventilation)
• Hypervolemia, Cl- expansion	
• Renal loss of H+:	
• edematous states (heart failure, nephrotic syndrome cirrhosis), hyperaldosteronism, excess ACTH, hypercortisolism, exogenous steroids, hyper-reninemia, severe hypokalemia, renal artery stenosis, bicarbonate administration.	

Selected etiologies of metabolic acidosis

• <u>Elevated</u> anion gap:
• Methanol intoxication
• Uremia
• Diabetic ketoacidosis[a], alcoholic ketoacidosis, starvation ketoacidosis
• Paraldehyde toxicity
• Isoniazid
• Lactic acidosis
▪ Type A: tissue ischemia
▪ Type B: Altered cellular metabolism
• Ethanol or ethylene glycol intoxication
• Salicylate intoxication
• <u>Normal</u> anion gap with an increase in [Cl-]
• GI loss of HCO_3-
▪ Diarrhea, ileostomy, proximal colostomy, ureteral diversion
• Renal loss of HCO_3-
▪ proximal RTA
▪ carbonic anhydrase inhibitor (acetazolamide)
• Renal tubular disease
▪ ATN
▪ Chronic renal disease
▪ Distal RTA
▪ Aldosterone inhibitors or absence
▪ NaCl infusion, TPN, NH_4+ administration.

Selected mixed and complex acid-base disturbances

Condition	Features	Selected situations
Respiratory alkalosis with metabolic alkalosis	↑in pH ↑ in HCO_3- ↓ in pCO_2	• Over ventilation of COPD • Cirrhosis with diuretics • Pregnancy with vomiting
Respiratory acidosis with metabolic acidosis	↓in pH ↑ in pCO_2 ↓ in HCO_3-	• Multi-organ failure • Intoxications • Cardiac arrest
Respiratory alkalosis with metabolic acidosis	pH is the normal range ↓ in pCO_2 ↓ in HCO_3-	• Sepsis • Salicylate toxicity • Renal failure with CHF or pneumonia • Advanced liver disease
Respiratory acidosis with metabolic alkalosis	pH is normal ↑ in pCO_2, and HCO_3-	• Severe hypokalemia • COPD with diuretics, vomiting, NG suction
Metabolic acidosis with metabolic alkalosis	pH and HCO_3- in the normal range	• Uremia or ketoacidosis by vomiting, NG suction, diuretics, etc.

Examples of ABGs

These examples are provided to assist students

Example 1:

You are asked to look at a 63-year-old lady who was admitted with breathing difficulties. Upon admission, the patient looks sleepy and is using 10L of oxygen via a mask. You conduct an ABG that shows the following results:

pH: 7.29 (Normal 7.35 – 7.45)

pCO_2: 9.2 kPa (4.7 – 6.0 kPa) OR 68.2 mmHg (35.2 – 45 mmHg)

pO_2: 7.0 kPa (11-13 kPa) OR 52.5 mmHg (82.5 – 97.5 mmHg)

HCO3–: 26 (22 – 26 mEq/L)

Base excess: +1 (-2 to +2)

Interpretation:

•The pO_2 is low, so the patient is in respiratory failure.

•The pH shows an acidosis and assesses the CO_2 to see if it contributes to the acidosis ($\uparrow CO_2$).

•In this given case scenario, the pCO_2 is raised significantly, which is likely to cause acidosis.

•In the context of low pO_2, a raised pCO_2 suggests the patient has type 2 respiratory failure.

•The HCO3 is normal, so the metabolic system does not contribute to the acidosis and is not compensating for the respiratory acidosis, suggesting that this is an acute derangement.

The base excess is within usual limits as there has been no major improvement in the quantity of HCO3–.

•If this respiratory acidosis is chronic, we would expect the kidneys to produce more HCO3– compensation, which would have resulted in an improved BE.

•Thus, it is **respiratory acidosis.**

•Respiratory acidosis was caused by type 2 respiratory dysfunction (failure of ventilation) due to elevated levels of CO_2 (hypercapnia).

- Confusion
- Reduced consciousness level
- Asterixis
- Bounding pulse

•Type 2 respiratory failure happens as a result of a ventilation failure. **The probable causes of this include those mentioned below:**

Potential causes of type 2 respiratory failure
•Increased resistance of airways – COPD/asthma
•Reduced respiratory effort – opioid effects (e.g. opiates)/brain stem lesions/extreme obesity
•Decreased lung area available for gas exchange – chronic bronchitis
•Neuromuscular complications – Guillain-Barré syndrome/motor-neurone disease
•Deformity – ankylosing spondylitis/flail chest.

Example 2:

A 17-year-old teen complains to A&E of a tense sensation in her chest, shortness of breath, and some tingling in her fingertips and around her lips. She has no relevant prior medical records and is not on any daily medications. The ABG is performed on the patient while breathing room air, and the findings are shown below:

•pH: 7.50 (Normal 7.35 – 7.45)
•pO_2: 14 kPa (11 – 13 kPa) OR 105 mmHg (82.5 – 97.5 mmHg)
•pCO_2: 3.4 kPa (4.7 – 6.0 kPa) OR 24 mmHg (35.2 – 45 mmHg)
•HCO3–: 22 (22 – 26 mEq/L)
•BE: +2 (-2 to +2)

Interpretation:

•A pO_2 of 14 kPa on-air is at the upper limit of normal, so the patient is not hypoxic.
•The pH of 7.49 is greater than average, and thus the patient is alkaline.
•The next step is to determine when the respiratory system leads to alkalosis (e.g. CO_2).
•CO_2 is poor, associated with alkalosis, but we now realize that the respiratory system responds to alkalosis, likely to be the whole cause.
•The next step is to look at HCO 3- and see if it still leads to alkalosis.

•HCO3- is normal, except in mixed respiratory and metabolic alkalosis, leaving us with isolated respiratory alkalosis.
•The bicarbonate is at the low end of its usual state, but this does not reflect compensation.
•Compensation will require a significantly larger reduction in HCO3−.
•Thus, it is a **respiratory alkalosis.**
•Respiratory alkalosis occurs because of increased ventilation, which can be caused by any of the following:

•**Anxiety – panic attack**
•**Pain – causing raised respiratory rate**
•**Hypoxia –sometimes seen after climbing to high altitude**
•**Pulmonary embolism**
•**Pneumothorax**
•**Iatrogenic (unnecessary mechanical ventilation).**

•A previously stable young person who had hyperventilation with peripheral and peri-oral tingling will have a reasonably common history of a panic attack (anxiety).
•As blood plasma becomes more alkaline, the concentration of freely ionized calcium, the biologically active portion of blood calcium, reduces (hypocalcemia).
•Since a portion of both hydrogen ions and calcium is tied to serum albumin, as blood becomes alkaline, bound hydrogen ions dissociate from albumin, release albumin to bind more calcium, and decrease the freely ionized portion of overall serum calcium that contributes to hypocalcemia.
•This hypocalcemia related to alkalosis is responsible for the paresthesia often seen with hyperventilation.

Example 3:
A 48-year-old male has been hospitalized with a one-day history of abdominal distention and extreme vomiting. A CT scan shows a large mass that causes intestinal obstruction. As part of the patient's examination, the surgical registrar demands that you review his blood gas (on the air) with the findings shown below:

pH: 7.50 (Normal 7.35 – 7.45)
pO_2: 12.8 kPa (11 – 13 kPa) OR 95.2 mmHg (82.5 – 97.5 mmHg)
pCO_2: 5.4 kPa (4.7 – 6.0 kPa) OR 41 mmHg (35.2 – 45 mmHg)
HCO3-: 29 (22 – 26 mEq/L)
BE: +3 (-2 to +2)

Interpretation:

- A pO_2 of 12.7 kPa on-air is normal, so the patient is not hypoxic.
- The pH of 7.50 is higher than expected, and thus the patient is alkaline.
- The next step is to confirm whether the respiratory system contributes to the alkalosis (e.g. ↓ CO_2).
- CO_2 is normal, not associated with alkalosis, but we now know that the respiratory system is not the source of this disruption.
- The next step is to check the HCO 3- and see if it explains the alkalosis.
- HCO3– is high, which is following by metabolic alkalosis.
- Value of base excess is raised, in keeping with an excess of HCO3–.
- The respiratory system may attempt to compensate for metabolic alkalosis by increasing pCO_2 (reducing ventilation), but for the time being, the respiratory system is likely to retain pCO_2 within the normal range.
- However, if the metabolic alkalosis persists, you expect the pCO_2 to rise and compensate for the metabolic alkalosis, as the respiratory center becomes progressively desensitized to the increasing levels of pCO_2.
- So it is a **metabolic alkalosis.**

- As a result of this patient's copious vomiting, large quantities of HCL were lost (e.g. stomach acid).
- This marks a net loss of H+ ions, meaning less H+ to bind to HCO3– and therefore freer HCO3– in the system.
- Due to vomiting, the patient is volume-depleted, resulting in the release of aldosterone and other mineralocorticoids, increasing HCO3– reabsorption by the kidneys, increasing the amount of free HCO3– in the serum.

Example 4:

You are called to examine a 59-year-old woman admitted to the acute medical unit at your hospital. The nurse tells you that she is out of breath even after providing 3 liters of oxygen through the nasal cannula. You take an arterial blood gas that shows the following results:
- pH: 7.30 (Normal 7.35 – 7.45)
- pO_2: 9.2 kPa (11 – 13 kPa) OR 68.2 mmHg (82.5 – 97.5 mmHg)
- pCO_2: 8.5 kPa (4.7 – 6.0 kPa) OR 63 mmHg (35.2 – 45 mmHg)
- HCO3-: 29 (22 – 26 mEq/L)
- BE: +4 (-2 to +2)

Interpretation:

- pO_2 at 9.2 kPa is poor, indicating that the patient is hypoxic.
- It is necessary to note that this pO_2 is much lower than you can expect for a patient with 3L of oxygen.
- The 3L oxygen flow rate through the nasal cannula is required to produce an inspired concentration (FiO_2) of about 32 percent. Therefore, you would expect pO_2 to be around 10 kPa less than that (e.g. 22 kPa).
- A 9.2 kPa pO_2 is therefore grossly abnormal and suggests severe hypoxia.
- The pH of 7.30 is lower than average, and thus the patient is acidic.
- The next task is to decide whether the respiratory system responds to acidosis (e.g. CO_2).
- CO_2 is greatly elevated, associated with acidosis (and type 2 respiratory failure), so we now know that the respiratory system is likely to cause this condition (or at least a contributor).

•The next move is to look at HCO 3-and see how it leads to acidosis.
•HCO3-is high, which is not associated with acidosis, so the metabolic pathway does not lead to acidosis.
•The increased HCO3– compensates for the low pH.
•Base excess is raised following the excess of HCO3–.
•There is an indication of metabolic compensation, as the HCO3– is raised significantly.
•So, it is **respiratory acidosis with metabolic compensation.**
•This patient has COPD and a consistently higher degree of CO_2.
•As a result, the metabolic system had time to prepare for more pH reductions by producing and preserving HCO3.
•This explains why the pH is only mildly acidic, despite a large rise in pCO_2.
•If this derangement in CO_2 were acute, there would not have been time for a compensatory response from the metabolic system.

Example 5:

A 90-year-old patient has fever, rigors, hypotension, and decreased urinary production. He seems lost and is unable to give any meaningful history. Basic paperwork was provided by the nursing home where the patient came from. You look at the available records and find that the district nurse changed this patient's catheter 24 hours earlier. The medical registrar starts with antibiotics, vigorous fluid resuscitation, and asks you to conduct arterial blood gas with the results. The patient was not on oxygen at that time.
pH: 7.29 (Normal 7.35 – 7.45)
pO_2: 12.3 kPa (11 – 13 kPa) OR 93 mmHg (82.5 – 97.5 mmHg)
pCO_2: 5.4 kPa (4.7 – 6.0 kPa) OR 41.2 mmHg (35.2 – 45 mmHg)
HCO3-: 15 (22 – 26 mEq/L)
BE: – 4 (-2 to +2)

Interpretation:

•pO_2 of 12.3 kPa is normal, except for hypoxia to induce confusion in the patient.

•The pH of 7.29 is unusually low, and thus the patient is highly acidic. The next task is to decide whether the respiratory system responds to acidosis (e.g. CO_2).

•CO_2 is normal, and so the respiratory system does not appear to contribute to acidosis.

•The next action is to look at the HCO 3- and see if it contributes to the acidosis.

•HCO3– is low, which is associated with acidosis, so the metabolic system is the source of this patient's acidosis.

•Base excess is minimal, consistent with the diagnosis of metabolic acidosis.

•There is no proof of respiratory compensation for this metabolic acidosis (e.g. by CO_2).).

•**Metabolic acidosis**

•**Urosepsis** – possibly due to clinical picture, and history of previous adjustments in the catheter.

•This patient appeared severely septic, with fever, hypotension, and signs of decreased end-organ perfusion (reduced urine output).

Reduced end-organ perfusion induces tissue hypoxia, which causes anaerobic respiration of cells to produce oxygen.

•Anaerobic respiration causes lactic acid as a by-product, resulting in the patient's serum's acidic pH, resulting in lactic acidosis.

Example 6:

A 22-year-old woman is taken to A&E by an ambulance with a 5-day history of vomiting and lethargy. When you start talking to the woman, you note that she is disoriented and seems clinically dehydrated. You cannot get any more details at the time, but the patient seems very distressed. You get IV access, send out a routine blood panel, and start some fluids. You ask the nurse to verify the patient's vitals, and she finds a raised respiratory rate, low blood pressure, and tachycardia. On the recommendation of the registrar, you conduct the ABG.

The ABG findings are shown below (the patient was breathing room air when this was taken).

pO_2: 13 kPa (11 – 13 kPa) OR 97.5 mmHg (82.5 – 97.5 mmHg)

pH: 7.3 (Normal 7.35 – 7.45)

pCO_2: 4.2 kPa (4.7 – 6.0 kPa) OR 30.7 mmHg (35.2 – 45 mmHg)

HCO3-: 13 (22 – 26 mEq/L)
BE: -4 (-2 to +2)

Interpretation:

•A pO_2 of 13 kPa is normal, excluding hypoxia as the cause of her confusion.
•The pH of 7.3 is abnormally low, and thus the patient's pH is acidic.
•The next move is to decide whether the respiratory system contributes to acidosis (e.g. ↑ CO_2).
•The CO_2 is low, and therefore, the respiratory system does not appear to be contributing to the acidosis.
•The next action is to look at the HCO3– and see if it contributes to the acidosis.
•HCO3– is low, which is compliant with acidosis, so the metabolic system is the cause of this patient's acidosis.
•Base excess is low, in keeping with metabolic acidosis.
•There is an indication of respiratory compensation for this metabolic acidosis (e.g. decreased CO_2).
•So, it is **metabolic acidosis with respiratory compensation.**
Capillary blood glucose: 32 mmol/L
Urinalysis for glucose +++ Ketones +++

Diabetic ketoacidosis (DKA)
•Diabetic ketoacidosis is initiated by a lack of insulin in the bloodstream.
•The shortage of insulin and the resulting rise in glucagon contributes to increased glucose production by the liver and an inability for the cells to use glucose.
•High blood glucose levels result in enhanced urinary glucose excretion, water intake and solutes, and osmotic diuresis (this directs to polyuria, dehydration, and polydipsia).
•Insulin deficiencies often result in the release of free fatty acids from adipose tissue (lipolysis) as the body has to generate sugar from a source other than glucose.

•These fatty acids are processed into ketone bodies to be used as a source of energy. Ketone bodies make the blood more acidic (metabolic acidosis).

•The body is trying to compensate for the metabolic acidosis by hyperventilating to blow off CO_2 and increase the pH.

•This hyperventilation, in its extreme form, can be seen as a Kussmaul respiration.

Example 7:

A 58-year-old man was found collapsed at home with a breathing rate of 6 breaths per minute and constricted pupils. An ambulance was called, and paramedics gave some naloxone. Upon arrival at A&E, his ABG revealed the following (not on oxygen at the time of the ABG):

pH: 7.31 (Normal 7.35 – 7.45)

pO_2: 7.8 kPa (11 – 13 kPa) OR 59 mmHg (82.5 – 97.5 mmHg)

pCO_2: 7.2 (4.7 – 6.0 kPa) OR 53 mmHg (35.2 – 45 mmHg)

HCO3-: 22 (22 – 26 mEq/L)

BE: +1 (-2 to +2)

Interpretation:

•pO_2 of 7.9 kPa is low, because we know the patient is in respiratory failure, so we need to know the CO_2 before we can determine which form of respiratory failure.

•The pH of 7.31 is abnormally low, and thus the patient's pH is acidic.

•The following step is to determine whether the respiratory system contributes to acidosis (e.g. ↑ CO_2).

•pCO_2 is elevated, and so the respiratory system responds to acidosis.

•Provided that pO_2 is low, we may assume that this gentleman has type 2 respiratory failure (low pO_2 and raised pCO_2)

•The next move is to take a look at HCO 3-.

•HCO3- is within the standard range.

•Given the relatively sudden onset of symptoms, there would have been no time for metabolic compensation.

Base excess is already in the normal range. Again, there is no metabolic compensation for this.

•So, there is **respiratory acidosis, and respiratory failure is type 2.**

•History shows that this man has overdosed on opioids, due to decreased consciousness, respiratory depression, and pupil constriction.
•Respiratory depression has progressed to hypoxia, hypercapnia, and eventually to respiratory acidosis.

Example 8:

A 77-year-old female was brought to the hospital 10 days ago with a broken femur. The orthopedic team has fixed the injury, and since then she has been an in-patient in the orthopedic ward for recovery. The patient's nurse is becoming more concerned as the patient's oxygen demands rise (currently, she is on 3L), and the patient is now tachypneic (respiratory rate 35). Besides, the patient has lately started moaning about calf pain.
You evaluate the patient and do an ABG that shows the following:
pH: 7.50 (Normal 7.35 – 7.45)
pO_2: 6 kPa (11 – 13 kPa) OR 45 mmHg (82.5 – 97.5 mmHg)
pCO_2: 3.0 kPa (4.7 – 6.0 kPa) OR 23.2 mmHg (35.2 – 45 mmHg)
HCO3- : 21 (22 – 26 mEq/L)
BE: 0 (-2 to +2)

Interpretation

•3 liters of oxygen are equivalent to 32%. Therefore, we would expect a pO_2 of roughly 22 kPa for a patient on this amount of oxygen.
•The 6 kPa pO_2 is therefore very low.
•The pH of 7.50 is abnormally high, and thus the patient is alkaline.
•The following step is to determine whether the respiratory system contributes to the alkalosis (e.g. ↓ CO_2).
•pCO_2 is minimal, and thus the respiratory system responds to alkalosis.
•The next move is to take a look at HCO3-.
•HCO3- is within the normal range, so the metabolic system does not contribute to the alkalosis and is not compensating for it.
•Base excess is within the normal range. Again, there is no metabolic compensation.
•**Respiratory alkalosis and type 1 respiratory failure.**

•From a previous history, this patient may have deep vein thrombosis and secondary pulmonary embolism.
•This has ensued in a growing need for oxygen.
•The patient is likely to be hyperventilated to preserve a sufficient level of oxygenation, so as a result, unnecessary levels of CO_2 are exhaled, leading to alkalosis.

Example 9

A 24-year-old student has just returned from Ghana. He has experienced extreme diarrhea in the last few days and has now been admitted to A&E. He is rather dehydrated and tachypnoeic on examination.
The ABG is conducted and shows the following:
pH: 7.32 (Normal 7.35 − 7.45)
pO_2: 14.7 kPa (11 − 13 kPa) OR 109.5 mmHg (82.5 − 97.5 mmHg)
pCO_2: 4.2 kPa (4.7 − 6.0 kPa) OR 30 mmHg (35.2 − 45 mmHg)
HCO3- : 13 (22 − 26 mEq/L)
BE: -4 (-2 to +2)

Interpretation

•pO_2 of 14.6 kPa is elevated and is likely to be due to hyperventilation.
•The pH of 7.32 is low, indicating that gentleman is acidic.
•We now need to look at pCO_2 to determine if this contributes (e.g. raised CO_2).
•pCO_2 is minimal, and thus the respiratory system does not lead to acidosis.
•, with this low CO_2, we might anticipate alkalosis, but we need to understand whether this is an effort by the respiratory system to compensate for metabolic acidosis. The next move is to have a look at the HCO3−
•HCO3− is low, which is consistent with our suspicion of metabolic acidosis.
•Base excess is also minimal, again in line with metabolic acidosis.
•So, it is **metabolic acidosis with respiratory compensation.**
•The patient is losing HCO3- via the gastrointestinal tract owing to diarrhea, contributing to metabolic acidosis.

•The respiratory system attempts to compensate by 'blowing off' carbon dioxide to create a respiratory alkalosis to neutralize the acidosis and bring the pH back into the normal range.

Example 10
A 60-year-old man is admitted to A&E with extreme central chest pain. He has a cardiac arrest as the nurses get him attached to the ECG. Luckily, the CPR started immediately, and after 6 minutes, the patient regained spontaneous circulation and began to breathe again.
Following this sequence of cases, the ABG (on 15L O_2) indicates the following:
pH: 7.14 (Normal 7.35 – 7.45)
pO_2: 9.5 kPa (Normal 11 – 13 kPa) OR 71.3 mmHg (82.5 – 97.5 mmHg)
pCO_2: 8.0 kPa (4.7 – 6.0 kPa) OR 60.7 mmHg (35.2 – 45 mmHg)
HCO3- : 15.2 (Normal 22 – 26 mEq/L)
BE: – 9.7 (-2 to +2)

Interpretation:
- kPa is a very poor value for pO_2, particularly in the perspective of 15L O_2. This demonstrates the presence of inadequate breathing, which is likely secondary to cardiac arrest.
- The pH of 7.14 is low, indicating that gentleman is acidic. We now need to look at pCO_2 to determine if this contributes (e.g. raised CO_2).
- pCO_2 is high, consistent with type 2 respiratory failure and also with respiratory acidosis. Again, this is likely to be secondary to poor breathing.
- The next move is to take a look at HCO3- .
- HCO3– is also low, indicating that the metabolic system also leads to acidosis.
- Base excess is minimal, again in line with metabolic acidosis.
- **Mixed respiratory acidosis and metabolic acidosis.**
- This patient had a cardiac arrest, which indicated a period of poor breathing and perfusion of the end organs.

- This eventually led to hypercapnia that triggered respiratory acidosis, in addition to the aggregation of anaerobic respiration-products (as a result of hypoxia and decreased end-organ perfusion) which caused metabolic acidosis.

Example 11

A 16-year-old woman presents drowsiness and vomiting in the hospital. They have no prior medical records, and have no daily prescription. The ABG is conducted on room air and shows the following:

- **pH**: 7.33 (Normal 7.35 – 7.45)
- **pO_2**: 14 (11 – 13 kPa) or 105 mmHg (82.5 – 97.5 mmHg)
- **pCO_2**: 3.2 (4.7 – 6.0 kPa) or 22.5 mmHg (35.2 – 45 mmHg)
- **HCO_3-**: 17 (22 – 26 mEq/L)

Interpretation:

Metabolic acidosis with respiratory compensation.

The underlying cause of metabolic acidosis, in this case, is *diabetic ketoacidosis*.

- pO_2 of 14 on room air is at the upper end of normal, such that the patient is not hypoxic.
- The pH of 7.33 is lower than average, and the patient's pH is also acidic.
- The next step is to decide if the respiratory system leads to acidosis (i.e., to CO_2).
- The CO_2 is low, eliminating the respiratory system as the cause of acidosis (as we would expect it to be increased, if this were the case).
- We recognize that the respiratory tract is NOT leading to acidosis and is, therefore, metabolic acidosis.
- The next phase is to look at the HCO3- to validate this.
- HCO3– is low, which is compatible with metabolic acidosis.
- We now know that the patient has metabolic acidosis, so we should look back at the CO_2 to see whether the respiratory system is trying to compensate for the metabolic condition.
- In this scenario, there is an indication of respiratory compensation when the CO_2 was reduced to normalize the pH.

- An important thing to consider here is that while the pH disruption tends to be comparatively mild, it should not be concluded that metabolic acidosis is, therefore, minor.
- The severity of metabolic acidosis is masked by the respiratory system's effort to compensate for decreased levels of CO_2.

Example 12

A 17-year-old patient complains to A&E of a tight sensation in her chest, shortness of breath, and some tingling in her fingertips and around her lips. She had no substantial medical records in the past and is not on any daily treatment. The ABG was done on the patient without oxygen administration

An **ABG** is performed and shows the following:
- **pH**: 7.49 (Normal values 7.35 – 7.45)
- **pO_2:** 105 mmHg (82.5 – 97.5 mmHg)
- **pCO_2:** 27 mmHg (35.2 – 45 mmHg)
- **HCO_3–** : 24 (22 – 26 mEq/L)

Interpretation
- pO_2 of 14 in room air is at the upper limit of normal, so the patient is not hypoxic.
- The pH of 7.49 is higher than normal, and therefore the patient is alkaline.
- The next step is to choose whether the respiratory system contributes to alkalosis (e.g. CO_2).
- CO_2 is low, which would be consistent with alkalosis, so we now know that the respiratory system contributes to alkalosis, if not the whole cause.
- The next step is to look at HCO3– and see if it also contributes to alkalosis.
- HCO3– is normal, excluding mixed respiratory and metabolic alkalosis, leaving us with isolated respiratory alkalosis.
- There is no evidence of respiratory alkalosis (which would involve lowered HCO3-), suggesting that this disturbance is relatively acute (as metabolic compensation requires a few days to develop).
- **Respiratory alkalosis without metabolic compensation.**

- In this case, respiratory alkalosis's underlying cause is a panic attack, with hyperventilation and peripheral and peri-oral tingling being classical features.

Example 13:

Mrs. Puffer is a 35-year-old female, just finishing the night shift. She has reported to the ED early in the morning with shortness of breath. She has cyanosis. She has had a productive cough for two weeks. She has 102.2, blood pressure of 110/76, heart rhythm of 108, respiration of 32, rapid and shallow. In both bases, the breathing sounds are diminished, with coarse rhonchi in the upper lobes. Chest X-ray refers to bilateral pneumonia.

ABG results are:
- pH = 7.44
- HCO3- = 24
- pO_2 = 54
- pCO_2 = 28

Interpretation:
- pCO_2 is low due to rapid breathing.
- pH is on the higher side of normal, so **compensated respiratory alkalosis**.
- pO_2 is also poor, presumably due to mucosal displacement of air in alveoli infected by pneumonia.

Example 14:
You are a critical care nurse going immediately to receive Mr. Sweet, a 24-year-old DKA (diabetic ketoacidosis) ED patient. The medical diagnosis says you expect to have acidosis. In the documents, you notice that his blood glucose was 780 on arrival. He was put on an insulin-infusion and obtained one bicarb amp. You are going to check the blood sugar level every hour by finger-prick test.

ABG results are:
- pH = 7.33
- HCO3- =12
- pO_2 = 89
- pCO_2 = 25

Interpretation
- The pH is acidic but still close to the normal range
- pCO_2 is 25 (low), which should make alkalosis.
- This is a **respiratory compensation for metabolic acidosis**.
- The underlying problem is, of course, **metabolic acidosis** due to ketones.

Conclusion

In human physiology, it is essential to address electrolytes, the main ingredient of body fluids, the extracellular fluid (ECF), and the overall body water (H_2O) content. Electrolytes are often better referred to collectively than separately because they are part of an interconnected biochemical system of H_2O and ion equilibrium. Kidney function and hormonal activity help to sustain electrolyte homeostasis.

These salts play a role in general functions of metabolic pathways, enzyme activation, acid-base balance, muscular-function regulation, and nervous-tissue contractions. Control of electrolyte levels is based on H_2O and pH balance, and is enacted by the renal tubules through active transport in the proximal convoluted tubules, osmosis, and passive diffusion. At the cellular level, sodium (NA+) and potassium (K+) levels are maintained by the Na-K-adenosine triphosphatase (ATPase) pump. The endocrine system affects the distal convoluted tubules through the renin-aldosterone system and circulating vasopressin and natriuretic peptides in body fluids.

The reference form for these electrolytes, rather than-HCO3−, is the photometry of flame emission. However, ion-selective electrodes (ISEs) are the most commonly used electrolyte analysis instruments in clinical laboratories. Only the ISE determines the free unbound ion; factors that influence binding and ionization may affect the precision of the measurements. ISEs comprise, or are covered by, a special substance that is more selective for a certain ion in solution, than for other ions. As the chosen ion comes into contact with the electrode, a difference in the potential may be seen relative to the reference electrode; this is measured as a change in the voltage due to the ionic action.

Turnaround Time (TAT) for urgent electrolyte-level test orders is weighed when selecting method platforms. It is normal to set the completion-time for immediate electrolyte-test requests at 15 minutes, while healthcare providers recommend a 5-minute TAT.

This is achievable by using point-of-care (POC) devices to accomplish this TAT. However, before developing this alternative, staff must consider different technological factors, such as issues of reliability of data.

POC devices can produce unreliable results due to variable levels of experience among testing staff, less care taken by certain testing-staff members, the effects of sample integrity, and the general assumption that simpler testing equates to error-proof results. With less control over the testing process, monitoring and handling POC electrolyte devices' errors can be more difficult than in the centralized laboratory-testing environment.

A procedure that does not induce hemolysis should be used to collect venous serum, lithium heparinized whole blood or plasma, heparinized whole arterial blood, release from muscle activity, or leakage erythrocytes. Heparinized plasma is the specimen of choice; it contains less K+, namely 0.3 to 0.7 mmol per L, than serum, due to platelet release during the coagulation process. Laboratories can also analyse electrolytes in body fluids such as urine, saliva, cerebrospinal fluid (CSF), and gastric fluids; specimens of these fluids are stable when kept in closed containers and analysed promptly. The specimen type may cause a consistent difference between direct and indirect ISE methods, especially when POC devices are used. This difference may occur due to the different ratios of the volume of anticoagulant-to-patient-specimen used in central laboratory testing, versus whole capillary blood that is tested in POC devices.

Several pre-analytical factors influence the electrolyte results, including anticoagulants, storage conditions, and hemolysis. Hemolysis of the blood produces a false rise in plasma K+ results by releasing intracellular K+; however, grossly hemolyzed specimens affect Na+ and Cl- levels of examination, due to dilution. The presence of excess anticoagulant when small amounts of blood are collected will similarly induce dilution, and wrongly lower plasma levels of Na+, and Cl- . Refrigeration of undivided whole blood may increase the intracellular release of K+ from erythrocytes.

With some anticoagulants, such as trisodium citrate ($Na_3C_6H_5O_7$) or ethylene-diamine-tetra-acetic acid (EDTA), chelate cations should be avoided in order to prevent a false decrease in plasma effects. Ammonium or sodium heparin can falsely add electrolytes to the result. Therefore, lithium heparin is the only anticoagulant recommended for the study of plasma electrolytes.

Analytical variables can also induce limitations. Flame emission and ISE devices that dilute the sample before electrode processing are indirect. The findings are impaired by hyperlipidemia or hyperproteinemia, because the large lipid or protein molecules that occur in unusually high amounts in those conditions displace some of the plasma's volumes within the dilution. For instance, if triglycerides or total protein are significantly elevated, the laboratory-tester may begin to experience interference. The effect of hyperlipidemia or hyperproteinemia is to lower the measured Na+ levels falsely, and sometimes the Cl- levels in the plasma, due to this dilutional effect. Direct systems should not dilute the material before analysis. Also, with normal H_2O plasma concentrations, a small variation in ionic activity can be calculated by direct and indirect ISE systems. Direct ISE systems typically have a conversion factor that results in concentrations equivalent to the reference process (flame photometry) for specimens with typical plasma H_2O levels.

Analytical limitations can be more severe than others in some methodologies. For example, a study of the POC system, which analyzes blood gases and electrolytes, reported substantially different amounts of Na+ than a benchtop analyzer in paired sample studies. The researchers recommend that critical decisions could safely be made based on POC K+ values but that Na+ results might not be as reliable.

The variation will also occur in the spectrophotometric method for determining the total CO_2 level, due to interfering chemicals that are absorbed in wavelengths which overlap with the wavelengths established for the test analysis.

The enzymatic/photometric method for total CO_2 may yield a false decrease in the results, due to turbidity production, which alters the enzymatic assay's reaction kinetics, and causes an initial increase in absorbance to give a falsely low total CO_2 value.

Turbidity may have resulted from paraproteins' precipitation, or an endogenous antibody that binds with an animal protein included in the assay reagents.

Reference ranges vary with populations, geographical locations, methods, and other conditions. A study suggests the need for separate reference intervals for neonates versus infants. The historical reference ranges regarding electrolytes being used by the National Institution of Health includes the following: Na+, 135 to 144 mmol/L; Cl-, 99 to 107 mmol/L; K+, 3.3 to 5.1 mmol/L; and total CO_2, 21 to 31 mmol/L. Developing specific standardized reference ranges and critical values can be useful in making clinical decisions.

Accurate electrolyte measurement and valid findings are essential to medical outcomes. It is necessary to use a well-maintained and well-qualified instrument; to pay critical attention to standard operating procedures; to refer to the information provided by the manufacturers of analyzers; and test methodologies to minimize pre-analytical, analytical, and post-analytical errors.

In conclusion, standardization of procedures for the processing, examination, and documentation of specimens, and adopting the best practices to validate cross-checking findings, is important for reducing laboratory errors.

Made in the USA
Las Vegas, NV
22 October 2024

10298239R00118